LIVER TUMORS - EPIDEMIOLOGY, DIAGNOSIS, PREVENTION AND TREATMENT

Edited by **Helen Reeves, Derek M. Manas** and **Rajiv Lochan**

Liver Tumors - Epidemiology, Diagnosis, Prevention and Treatment
http://dx.doi.org/10.5772/56514
Edited by Helen Reeves, Derek M. Manas and Rajiv Lochan

Contributors

Radu Ion Badea, Simona Ioanitescu, Radu Badea, Mariana Mihaila, Laurentiu Micu, Tetsuya Nakatsura, Yu Sawada, Kazuya Ofuji, Mayuko Sakai, Alejandro Serrablo, Luis Tejedor, Jose M. Ramia-Ángel, Hueseyin Bektas, Arndt Vogel, Nora Schweitzer, Charing Ching Ning Chong

Published by InTech

Janeza Trdine 9, 51000 Rijeka, Croatia

Publishing Process Manager Ana Pantar
Technical Editor InTech DTP team
Cover InTech Design team

Additional hard copies can be obtained from orders@intechopen.com

Liver Tumors - Epidemiology, Diagnosis, Prevention and Treatment, Edited by Helen Reeves, Derek M. Manas and Rajiv Lochan
p. cm.
ISBN 978-953-51-1070-5

For EU product safety concerns:
IN TECH d.o.o., Prolaz Marije Krucifikse Kozulić 3, 51000 Rijeka, Croatia,
info@intechopen.com or visit our website at intechopen.com.

Meet the editors

Helen Reeves Graduated from Nottingham Medical school in 1990 before moving to Newcastle-upon-Tyne in 1991. She completed her basic training in Hepatology in parallel with basic science research, being awarded a PhD studying signaling pathways central to liver fibrogenesis in 2001. She subsequently completed 3 years training as a postdoctoral scientists with Professor Scott Friedman at Mount Sinai Medical School in New York, focusing largely on molecular pathogenesis of cancers, before returning to Newcastle as a Senior Clinician Scientist in 2004. She is presently the clinical hepatology lead for care of patients with HCC in Northern England, while academically she heads a team of 10 basic scientists and students in the Northern Institute for Cancer Research at Newcastle University.

Professor Derek M. Manas is a hepatobiliary and transplant surgeon who trained in Cape Town, South Africa and completed fellowships at 'Johns Hopkins - USA' and 'Paul-Brousse, Paris'. He joined the NHS at the Freeman Hospital in 1994 and attained a personal chair in Transplantation in 2007. He has been instrumental in successfully developing three super-regionally funded transplant programmes in the North East of England (Liver, Pancreas and Islets) as well as most recently the UK's first 'Institute for Transplantation' in Newcastle. He is a member or chair of a number of national committees and has a well established national and international research reputation in primary liver cancer, radio-frequency ablation of liver tumours and liver transplantation for primary liver cancer.

Rajiv Lochan is Senior Fellow in HPB & Liver Transplant surgery at the Freeman Hospital, Newcastle-upon-Tyne. He completed basic training from the University of Mysore and subsequently worked as a Research Fellow in Newcastle where he developed his research interests into the role of DNA damage repair mechanisms in the development of HPB cancers. He subsequently completed Higher Specialist Training in General, HPB and Abdominal Transplantation Surgery in 2012. His clinical research interests include improving outcomes from the management of Liver, pancreatic and retroperitoneal tumours, Liver Transplantation surgery and Acute pancreatitis. In the middle of 2013, he is due to commence a Fellowship at Queen Mary's Hospital, Hong Kong furthering his interest in HCC management and Living Donor Liver Transplantation.

Contents

Preface

Tumours of the liver are frequently benign incidental findings. If malignant, however, the prognosis for those affected is often poor. Malignancies include those which have metastasized to the liver from elsewhere, reflecting advanced stage cancers where cure is rarely possible. Similarly, primary liver cancer frequently complicates chronic liver disease, which further limits therapeutic options even for disease presenting at a relatively early stage. In fact, primary liver cancer remains one of the few types of cancer where annual mortality figures and incidence are both similar and increasing, reflecting a relative lack of progress in either prevention of the disease or its treatment. Despite these dismal data, there are signs that change is imminent. Surgery remains the goal for treatment of metastatic or primary liver tumours, and advances in surgical techniques as well as tumour 'downstaging' offer potential cure to small but ever increasing numbers of individuals. Successful treatment of viral hepatitis has been rewarded in some parts of the globe with falling incidence of primary cancers, while novel means of prevention are also emerging. Imaging modalities have also advanced over the last two to three decades, facilitating surveillance programmes and earlier stage detection of tumours. Medical therapies have markedly improved survival of patients with liver metastases and while the impact of medical therapies for primary liver cancers remains relatively disappointing, small but highly significant advances have been made. In this book, an overview of different liver tumours is presented, focusing particularly on recent developments. As well as an update on epidemiology and risk factors for primary liver cancer, the role of contrast enhanced ultrasound is reviewed, as are the very important roles of anti-viral therapy and the exciting potential of immunotherapy. Management of both primary and metastatic cancers from a surgical perspective is comprehensively covered, including guidance for post therapeutic follow-up. This book serves as an accurate up to date guide for a common and increasing clinical problem. The book will be relevant for all researchers and practitioners involved in the care of patients with liver tumours.

Editor:
Helen Reeves
Newcastle University, UK

Co-editors:
Derek M. Manas
Institute of Transplantation, Newcastle upon Tyne, NHS Hospital Trust, UK

Rajiv Lochan
Freeman Hospital, Newcastle upon Tyne, UK

Chapter 1

Epidemiology and Risk Factors

Nora Schweitzer and Arndt Vogel

Additional information is available at the end of the chapter

http://dx.doi.org/10.5772/55908

1. Introduction

1.1. Epidemiology

Worldwide, hepatocellular carcinoma (HCC) is is the fifth most common cancer in men and the seventh in women (Figure 1). Because of impaired treatment options and late diagnosis in many cases, mortality is almost as high as the incidence rate (mortality: incidence rate 0.93). Worldwide, it is the third most frequent cause of tumour-related deaths. In the year 2008, 748,300 new HCCs and 695,900 deaths have been registered (http://www.iarc.fr/). Almost 85% of all cases occur in the developing countries (Figure 1). Regions with a high incidence are Eastern and South-Eastern Asia and Middle and Western Africa. More than a half of all new HCC are diagnosed in China, resulting in an incidence of 35.2/ 100000 inhabitants. While North America, Australia and Northern Europe belong to the low-incidence areas, the incidence is significantly higher in Southern Europe (10.5 per 100,000) (Figure 2).

The HCC incidence increases with age [1-3]. Only in regions with high hepatitis B virus (HBV) infection rate, e.g. China, are patients younger at diagnosis, presenting at 55-59 years of age. In contrast, in Japan, where chronic hepatitis C virus (HCV) infection is the most important risk factor for HCC, the peak age is between 70 and 79 years. In Europe and North America most patients are between 60 and 65 years old at diagnosis [4].

In most countries, HCC represents 80% - 90% of all primary liver tumours. An exception is the Khon Kaen region of Thailand, which is known for its high incidence rates of 88/100,000 for men and 35.4/100,000 for women. In this area, the main tumour entity is cholangiocellular carcinoma caused by endemic infestation with liver flukes [5].

Worldwide, the incidence of HCCs is increasing. In Europe and USA, a peak is expected in 2020. In particular, frequent HCV infections during the 50th and the 60th are made responsible for that fact. During the last two decades, the mortality rates have increased in some European

Countries (e.g. Germany, Austria) and in the US, where the mortality has risen by 40% from 1994 to 2004 [6]. On the other hand, some countries, e.g. France and Italy, have shown a strong increase of mortality-rates in the mid-nineties and a decline thereafter [7].

In almost all populations, more men than women are affected. Men/women ratios of 2:1 to 4:1 in high-risk areas are registered. Certainly, the fact that men are more often exposed to risk factors partly accounts for the higher incidence for men. However, as gender differences can be reproduced in mouse experiments, hormonal changes are likely to influence hepatocarcinogenesis as well. One possible mechanism is that androgens enhance DNA damage and oxidative stress during hepatocarcinogenesis [8]. Furthermore, the inhibition of interleukin-6 production in Kupffer cells by estrogens may be relevant in gender-specific hepatocarcinogenesis [9]. Recently, it was shown that the transcription factor foxa1/2 protects female mice from HCC while promoting HCC in male mice [10]. All these results indicate that there exist gender specific mechanisms in hepatocarcinogenesis and that the higher incidence of HCC in men is not restricted to the exposure to risk factors.

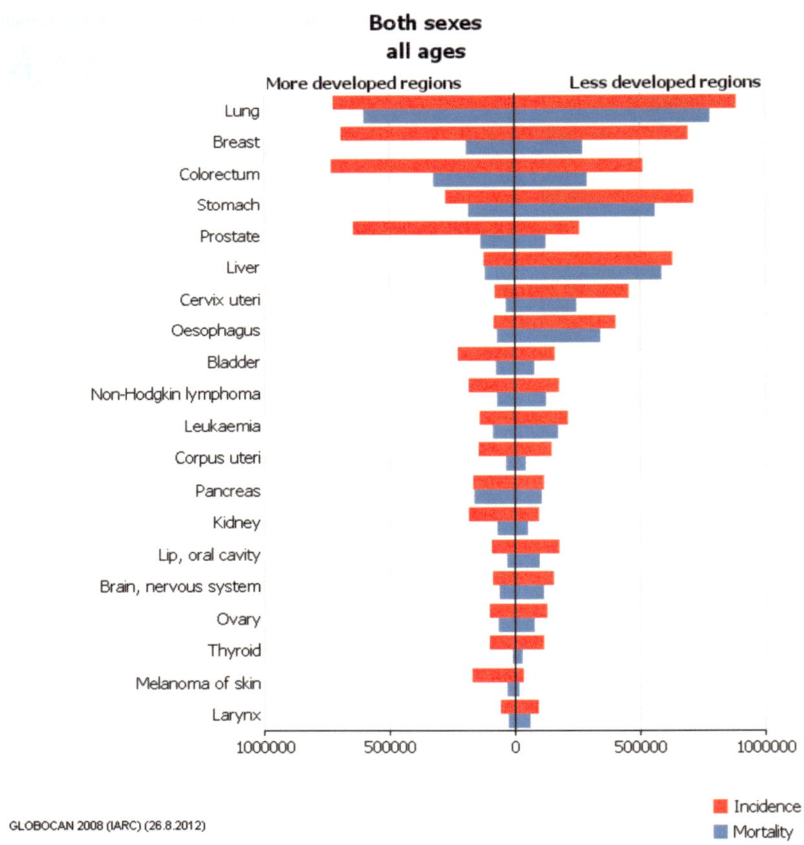

Figure 1. Cancer Incidence and Mortality Worldwide, Both Sexes

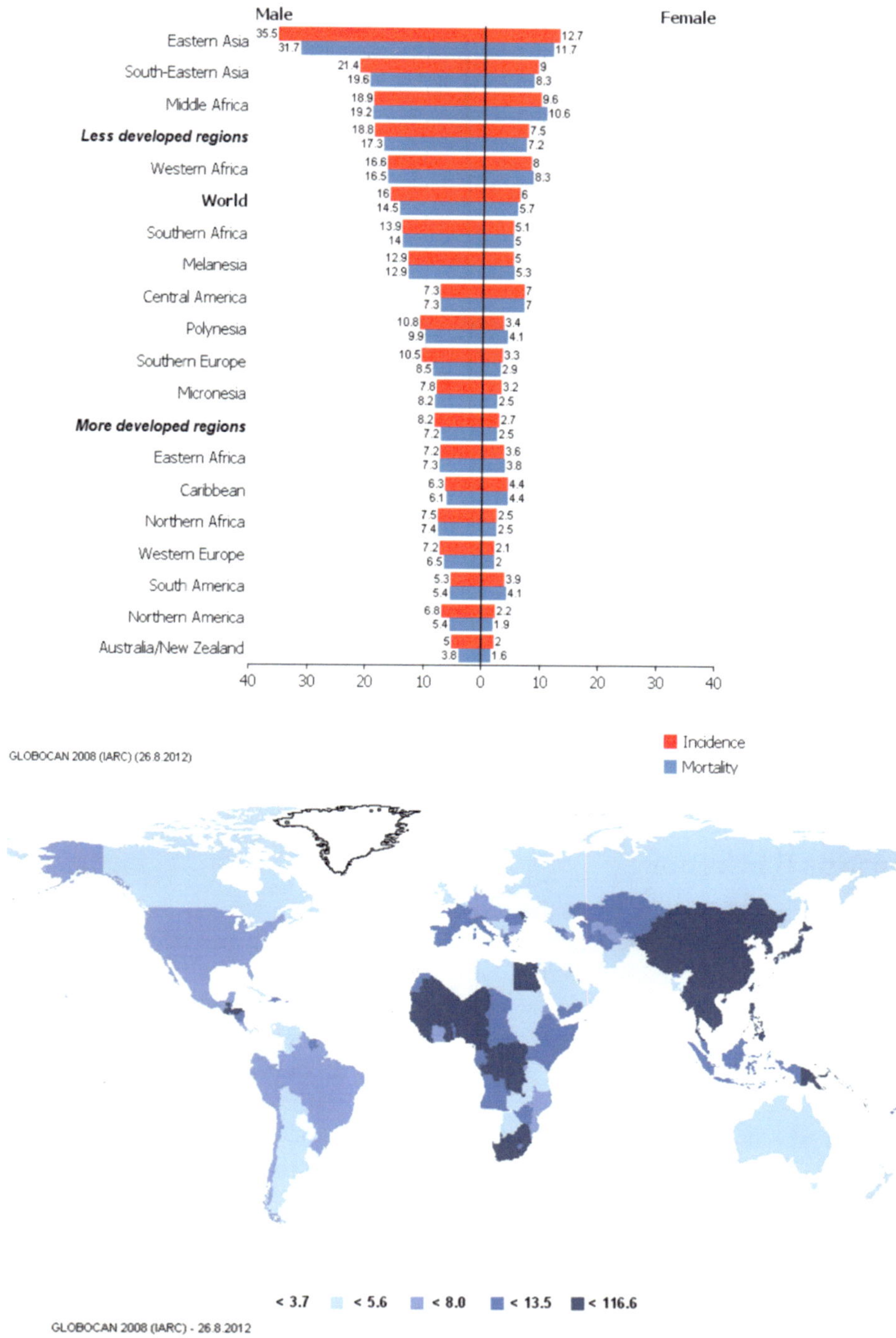

Figure 2. Incidence and Mortality of HCC Worldwide (per 100,000)

2. Risk factors

In more than 70% of all cases, HCC develops in patients with advanced liver cirrhosis. In 90%, the responsible risk factor is known. The main risk factors for liver cirrhosis and HCC strongly depend on the geographic region. Worldwide, the most important risk factors are viral hepatitis, alcohol und aflatoxin exposure (Table 1). 54% of all HCC can be attributed to hepatitis B and 31% to hepatitis C. Interestingly, signs of advanced cirrhosis such as portal hypertension correlate with the development of HCC.

Region	M/F	Risk factors (%)			
		HCV	HBV	Alcohol	others
Europe	6,7/ 2,3	60-70	10-15	20	10
North America	4,1/ 2,3	50-60	20	20	10 (NASH)
Asia and Africa		20	70	10	10 (Aflatoxin)
Asia	21,6/ 8,2				
China	23/ 9,6				
Japan	20,6/ 7,8	70	10-20	10	10
Africa	1,6/ 5,3				
World	16/ 6	31	54	15	

Table 1. Distribution of Risk Factors by Geographic Region (adapted from EASL-EORTC Clinical Practice Guidelines 2012 [11])

3. Hepatitis B infection

Overall, 400 million people are infected with HBV. While in Asia and Africa up to 70% of all HCC patients suffer from HBV infection, hepatitis B is found in only 20% as the underlying risk factor in Europe and USA. Worldwide, about 50% of all HCC are due to HBV infection. In areas with a high incidence of hepatitis B, especially in Asia, vertical transmission is most common and subsequently, 90% of infected newborns develop chronic HBV infection. Countries with a high incidence of HBV infections significantly reduced the rate of new diagnosis by routine vaccination of newborns [12]. In low-incidence areas, HBV most often is transmitted in the adulthood via sexual or parenteral contacts [13]. In this population, the infection may resolve spontaneously in up to 90% of cases.

Up to 25% of all chronically infected individuals will eventually develop HCC [14]. HCC does not exclusively occur in cirrhotic livers, but also in non-cirrhotic livers of nearly 30% of high viremic patients. The risk for the development of HCC of HBV infected patients is elevated to 5 to 100fold. Main risk factors are long-term high viremia (>2000 IU/ml) (Figure 3), high aminotransferases, positive HBeAg and infection with HBV genotype C [15;16]. As patient related risk factors, male gender, more than 40 years of age, positive family history for HCC,

http://dx.doi.org/10.5772/55908

migration background from hyperendemic areas, co-infection with hepatitis D virus, HIV or HCV and exposure to alcohol or aflatoxins were identified.

The molecular mechanisms of hepatitis B virus-induced hepatocarcinogenesis are not completely understood. Ongoing inflammation and cell damage lead to an increase of cell turnover, which finally results in an accumulation of genetic alterations. These may also be caused by chromosomal integrations of HBV, which can be found in up to 80% of all HBV-related HCC. Furthermore, some viral proteins can transactivate growth factors and proto-oncogenes like c-MYC.

Patients with chronic hepatitis B or hepatitis B/D co-infection should be treated according to current guidelines. Treatment options for HBV-infected patients are nucleoside/nucleotide analogues or interferon alpha. Sustained HBV suppression can prevent the progression to cirrhosis and hence lower the risk for HCC. Once cirrhosis is established, the preventive potential of antiviral drugs in chronic hepatitis B has not been robustly demonstrated. Ultrasound examination every six month +/- AFP measurement for HCC screening in patients at risk is strongly recommended.

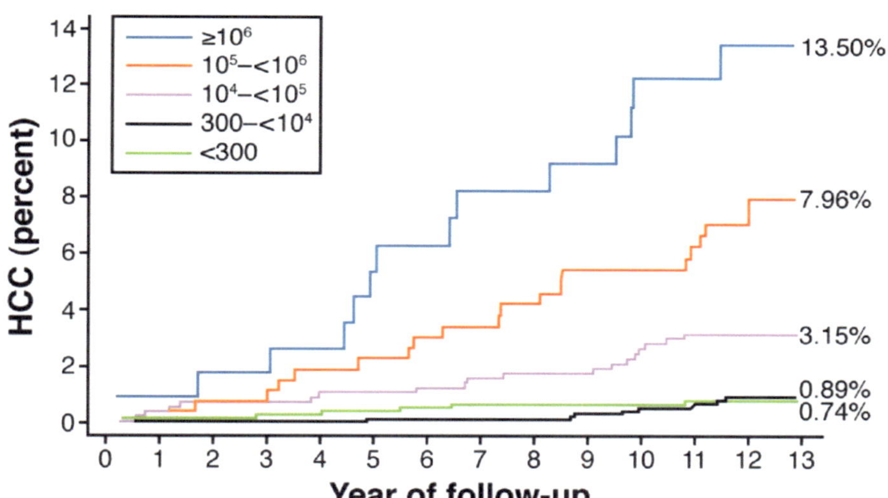

Figure 3. Association of Serum Level HBV DNA and the Development of HCC (from Hashem B El-Serag, Gastroenterology 2012, adapted from Chen CJ. JAMA 2006 [17]

4. Hepatitis C infection

Similar to hepatitis B, patients with hepatitis C are at higher risk to develop HCC. Worldwide, over 180 million people are infected [2% of the global population) and about 30% of HCC are HCV-related.

In the late 1920s, the first HCV infections occurred in Japan. Not before the 1940s, it spread in Southern Europe and in the 1960s and 1970s many people in North America were infected, mainly due to intravenous drug use but also via medical procedures. The virus contaminated national blood supplies and circulated until the late 1980s. Nowadays, the highest prevalence of HCV is found in Egypt, being 9% countrywide and up to 50% in certain areas [18]. Recent data suggest that HCC occurs decades after infection and that the risk is strongly elevated in patients older than 65 years compared to younger patients [19]. Thus, the temporal distribution of the HCV-endemic is one reason for the differences in the incidence rates HCC in different areas.

HCV infection is chronic in most patients. It goes along with a variable degree of hepatic inflammation and results in cirrhosis in 10-40%. At the stage of cirrhosis, HCC is the main complication and the main cause of death. Compared to non-infected individuals, the risk for HCC is 17fold elevated. In contrast to HBV, in HCV infected patients, tumours occur primarily in the cirrhotic liver. The risk per year to develop HCC in patients with HCV-related cirrhosis is 5%. It increases when additional risk factors are present, e.g. genotype 1b, alcohol or cigarette consumption or a co-infection with HBV or HIV [20,21].

In contrast to HBV, HCV cannot integrate into the human genome. Instead, apparently several viral proteins have tumorigenic effects. In rodents, it has been shown that overexpression of NS3 induces HCC. Patients with HCV infection are recommended to obtain treatment according to current guidelines. Treatment options for hepatitis C are interferon alpha, ribavirin and more recently also protease inhibitors. In patients with sustained response, HCC incidence is markedly reduced [22]. Excepted to this protective effect are patients with evident cirrhosis. Thus, screening for HCC via ultrasound and eventually AFP measurement are recommended every six months.

5. Alcohol, coffee and tobacco

Alcohol alone probably is not carcinogen. However, excessive alcohol intake is one of the most frequent reasons for liver cirrhosis and thus an important risk factor for HCC. Recent epidemiologic case control studies suggest that not only alcohol (in 10% of all HCC) but also tobacco consumption (in almost 50% of all HCC) is a relevant cofactor for hepatocarcinogenesis [23]. Particularly in patients with HCV, and to a lesser extent, with HBV infection, the risk to develop HCC increases significantly already with moderate alcohol and tobacco consumption [24,25]. A large retrospective study of 36,000 liver cancer related deaths in Chinese demonstrated a dose-dependent elevation of the risk to die of liver cancer in cigarette-smokers. Main risk factor in this population was HBV. While patients who smoked less than 20 cigarettes per day had a 32% increase of risk compared to nonsmokers, patients with a cigarette-consumption of 20 or more per day had a 50% increase of risk [26]. However, the study provided no information about simultaneous alcohol consumption. In contrast, numerous epidemiologic studies showed a protective effect of coffee on the development of liver cirrhosis and HCC [27]. To date, the underlying mechanisms are not yet understood [27,28].

http://dx.doi.org/10.5772/55908

6. Metabolic syndrome

Prospective and retrospective studies identified diabetes mellitus as an important risk factor for the development of HCC, independent from the underlying liver disease [29,30]. Non-alcoholic liver disease (NAFLD) and non-alcoholic steatohepatitis (NASH) are more and more regarded as a hepatic manifestation of the metabolic syndrome, which is characterized by the combination of obesity, insulin resistance or diabetes, dyslipidemia and arterial hypertension. In US and other western countries, NAFLD is the most common liver disease of adults. However, only 20% of the individuals with NAFLD present with steatohepatitis, while the majority only have steatosis. Isolated steatosis of the liver probably has no effect on liver-related mortality [31-33].

NAFLD is found in 75% of patients with diabetes and 90% of obese patients with a body mass index of more than 40kg/m^2. Based on a cohort study of 900000 Americans, it has been proposed that men with a body mass index of 35kg/m2 or above have a 4.5 times higher risk for dying from liver cancer compared to men with a normal BMI. Similarly, a meta-analysis revealed a relative risk of liver cancer of 117% for overweight and 189% for obese persons [34]. The risk for developing HCC is less in NAFLD than in Hepatitis C but due to the increasing prevalence, NALFD and NASH are nowadays more often identified as underlying risk factor in patients with newly diagnosed HCC than HCV infection [35].

Currently, NAFLD is still believed to be underestimated as underlying risk factor for HCC. One reason is that once cirrhosis is established, key elements of NASH as hepatocellular lipid accumulation, ballooning injury and necroinflammation are no longer detectable in the cirrhotic liver [36]. Accordingly, the underlying disease in cryptogenic cirrhosis may be NAFLD in a considerable proportion of cases. Furthermore, NAFLD and other risk factors for HCC can occur simultaneously but mostly the second risk factor, e.g. HCV, is counted as the responsible risk factor. An alarming sign is that tumours develop in non-cirrhotic livers in up to 50%, meaning that the population at risk is higher than originally estimated [37].

Until now, neither a treatment for NAFLD or NASH, nor a strategy to prevent HCC in NAFLD has been established. A major focus certainly will be put on the insulin resistance of NAFLD patients. The results of several retrospective studies and meta-analyses suggest a preventive role of metformin in diabetic patients, while sulfonylurea drugs and insulin seem to facilitate the development of cirrhosis [38-40].

7. Aflatoxins

One important risk factor for HCC is the exposure to aflatoxins in some geographic regions. The toxins of the fungus aspergillus flavus and aspergillus parasiticus are ubiquitous in parts of Africa and Asia. By contamination of corn, nuts and legumes they enter the food chain and affect the broad population. Aflatoxin by itself is biologically inactive and displays its full effect only after ingestion by activation to aflatoxin B1-8,9-epoxide. The electrophil epoxide binds covalently to DNA bases and thereby becomes mutagenic. Epidemiologic investigations revealed frequent mutations in the tumour suppressor p53 in these patients. Simultaneous exposition of aflatoxins and HBV infection results in a more than additive risk for HCC.

8. Host factors

In first place, hemochromatosis and hereditary tyrosinemia type 1 (HT1) are genetic diseases associated with HCC. Hemochromatosis is an autosomal recessive disorder due to a mutation in the HFE gene. It is characterized by an increased intestinal absorption of iron, resulting in an accumulation and deposition of iron in organs like liver, pancreas, skin, heart and pituitary. In the liver, progressive accumulation of iron leads to fibrosis and cirrhosis and promotes the development of HCC. Affected patients are at 20fold higher risk to develop HCC.

HT1 is an autosomal recessive inherited disease, which is characterized by progressive liver disease and damage of the proximal renal tubular cells. It is caused by a deficiency of the enzyme fumarylacetoacetate hypdrolase (FAH), resulting in an accumulation of the substrate fumarylacetoacetate (FAA). FAA causes oxidative damage and is mutagenic. Untreated, the lifespan is dramatically shortened. Patients die from acute or chronic liver failure or from HCC in the first two decades of life. Therapeutically, nitisinone (or NTBC), an inhibitor of the enzyme 4-OH phenylpyruvate dioxygenase (HPD) can prevent accumulation of FAA.

Beside disease-causing mutations, there is growing evidence for a genetic susceptibility for HCC. In line with this, the risk to develop HCC is higher in individuals with a family history of HCC [32]. A predisposing effect is being suggested for numerous single nucleotide polymorphisms (SNP). A relationship between the carriage of a SNP and HCC in the investigated cohorts was demonstrated for SNPs in various genes, for example HFE (rs1800562), UGT1A7 (rs17868323 and rs11692021), MDM2 (rs2279744), IL-1B (rs1143627), MnSOD (rs4880), TNFalpha (G-308), EGF (61*G, rs4444903), cyclin D1 (G870A) [41]. The common variant rs738409 C>G in the adiponutrin/patatin-like phospholipase-3 (PNPLA3) protein sequence has consistently shown to be associated with hepatic steatosis, advanced fibrosis and a higher incidence of cirrhosis in patients with alcoholic [42] and non alcoholic fatty liver disease [43] and chronic HCV infection [44]. In patients with alcohol induced cirrhosis it is a risk factor for the development of HCC [45].

9. Conclusion

Worldwide, HCC incidence is increasing. The most important risk factors for HCC are hepatitis B and C, alcohol consumption and aflatoxin exposure. The increase of HCC in patients with steatohepatitis is alarming and is likely to be a major problem in developed countries in the future. Most HCC develop in cirrhotic livers but particularly in patients with hepatitis B or NASH, it can also occur in non-cirrhotic livers. Screening programs are important for all patients with liver cirrhosis to detect HCC in an early stage.

Author details

Nora Schweitzer and Arndt Vogel*

*Address all correspondence to: vogel.arndt@mh-hannover.de

Department of Gastroenterology, Hepatology and Endocrinology, Hannover Medical School, Germany

References

[1] El-Serag, H. B, & Mason, A. C. *Rising incidence of hepatocellular carcinoma in the United States.* N Engl J Med, (1999)., 745-750.

[2] *National Environmental Policy Act of 1969,* in *U.S.C.*(1994)., 102-105.

[3] Ekstedt, M, et al. *Long-term follow-up of patients with NAFLD and elevated liver enzymes.* Hepatology, (2006)., 865-873.

[4] Tanaka, H, et al. *Declining incidence of hepatocellular carcinoma in Osaka, Japan, from 1990 to 2003.* Ann Intern Med, (2008)., 820-826.

[5] El-Serag, H. B, & Rudolph, K. L. *Hepatocellular carcinoma: epidemiology and molecular carcinogenesis.* Gastroenterology, (2007)., 2557-2576.

[6] Jemal, A, et al. *Cancer statistics, 2008.* CA: a cancer journal for clinicians, (2008)., 71-96.

[7] Bosetti, C, et al. *Trends in mortality from hepatocellular carcinoma in Europe, 1980-2004.* Hepatology, (2008)., 137-145.

[8] Ma, W. L, et al. *Androgen receptor is a new potential therapeutic target for the treatment of hepatocellular carcinoma.* Gastroenterology, (2008). e1-5., 947-955.

[9] Naugler, W. E, et al. *Gender disparity in liver cancer due to sex differences in MyD88-dependent IL-6 production.* Science, (2007)., 121-124.

[10] Li, Z, et al. *Foxa1 and Foxa2 are essential for sexual dimorphism in liver cancer.* Cell, (2012)., 72-83.

[11] European Association For The Study Of TheL., R. European Organisation For, and C. Treatment Of, *EASL-EORTC clinical practice guidelines: management of hepatocellular carcinoma.* J Hepatol, (2012)., 908-943.

[12] Chang, M. H, et al. *Universal hepatitis B vaccination in Taiwan and the incidence of hepatocellular carcinoma in children. Taiwan Childhood Hepatoma Study Group.* N Engl J Med, (1997)., 1855-1859.

[13] El-Serag, H. B. *Epidemiology of viral hepatitis and hepatocellular carcinoma.* Gastroenterology, (2012). e1., 1264-1273.

[14] Ganem, D, & Prince, A. M. *Hepatitis B virus infection--natural history and clinical consequences.* N Engl J Med, (2004). , 1118-1129.

[15] Chen, C. J, et al. *Risk of hepatocellular carcinoma across a biological gradient of serum hepatitis B virus DNA level.* JAMA : the journal of the American Medical Association, (2006). , 65-73.

[16] Yu, M. W, et al. *Hepatitis B virus genotype and DNA level and hepatocellular carcinoma: a prospective study in men.* Journal of the National Cancer Institute, (2005). , 265-272.

[17] Chen, C. J, et al. *Risk of hepatocellular carcinoma across a biological gradient of serum hepatitis B virus DNA level.* JAMA, (2006). , 65-73.

[18] Kamal, S. M, & Nasser, I. A. *Hepatitis C genotype 4: What we know and what we don't yet know.* Hepatology, (2008). , 1371-1383.

[19] Asahina, Y, et al. *Effect of aging on risk for hepatocellular carcinoma in chronic hepatitis C virus infection.* Hepatology, (2010). , 518-527.

[20] Donato, F, et al. *Alcohol and hepatocellular carcinoma: the effect of lifetime intake and hepatitis virus infections in men and women.* Am J Epidemiol, (2002). , 323-331.

[21] Lok, A. S, et al. *Incidence of hepatocellular carcinoma and associated risk factors in hepatitis C-related advanced liver disease.* Gastroenterology, (2009). , 138-148.

[22] Lok, A. S, et al. *Maintenance peginterferon therapy and other factors associated with hepatocellular carcinoma in patients with advanced hepatitis C.* Gastroenterology, (2011). quiz e12., 840-849.

[23] Trichopoulos, D, et al. *Hepatocellular carcinoma risk factors and disease burden in a European cohort: a nested case-control study.* Journal of the National Cancer Institute, (2011). , 1686-1695.

[24] Ascha, M. S, et al. *The incidence and risk factors of hepatocellular carcinoma in patients with nonalcoholic steatohepatitis.* Hepatology, (2010). , 1972-1978.

[25] Chuang, S. C, et al. *Interaction between cigarette smoking and hepatitis B and C virus infection on the risk of liver cancer: a meta-analysis.* Cancer epidemiology, biomarkers & prevention : a publication of the American Association for Cancer Research, cosponsored by the American Society of Preventive Oncology, (2010). , 1261-1268.

[26] Chen, Z. M, et al. *Smoking and liver cancer in China: case-control comparison of 36,000 liver cancer deaths vs. 17,000 cirrhosis deaths.* Int J Cancer, (2003). , 106-112.

[27] Bravi, F, et al. *Coffee drinking and hepatocellular carcinoma risk: a meta-analysis.* Hepatology, (2007). , 430-435.

[28] Larsson, S. C, & Wolk, A. *Coffee consumption and risk of liver cancer: a meta-analysis.* Gastroenterology, (2007). , 1740-1745.

[29] Larsson, S. C, & Wolk, A. *Overweight, obesity and risk of liver cancer: a meta-analysis of cohort studies.* British journal of cancer, (2007). , 1005-1008.

[30] Wang, C, et al. *Increased risk of hepatocellular carcinoma in patients with diabetes mellitus: a systematic review and meta-analysis of cohort studies.* International journal of cancer. Journal international du cancer, (2012). , 1639-1648.

[31] Rafiq, N, et al. *Long-term follow-up of patients with nonalcoholic fatty liver.* Clin Gastroenterol Hepatol, (2009). , 234-238.

[32] Turati, F, et al. *Family history of liver cancer and hepatocellular carcinoma.* Hepatology, (2012). , 1416-1425.

[33] Calle, E. E, et al. *Overweight, obesity, and mortality from cancer in a prospectively studied cohort of U.S. adults.* N Engl J Med, (2003). , 1625-1638.

[34] Larsson, S. C, & Wolk, A. *Overweight, obesity and risk of liver cancer: a meta-analysis of cohort studies.* Br J Cancer, (2007). , 1005-1008.

[35] 35. Ertle, J, et al. *Non-alcoholic fatty liver disease progresses to hepatocellular carcinoma in the absence of apparent cirrhosis.* International journal of cancer. Journal international du cancer, (2011). , 2436-2443.

[36] Poonawala, A, Nair, S. P, & Thuluvath, P. J. *Prevalence of obesity and diabetes in patients with cryptogenic cirrhosis: a case-control study.* Hepatology, (2000). Pt 1): , 689-692.

[37] Baffy, G, Brunt, E. M, & Caldwell, S. H. *Hepatocellular carcinoma in non-alcoholic fatty liver disease: An emerging menace.* J Hepatol, (2012).

[38] Hassan, M. M, et al. *Association of diabetes duration and diabetes treatment with the risk of hepatocellular carcinoma.* Cancer, (2010). , 1938-1946.

[39] Chen, H. P, et al. *Metformin decreases hepatocellular carcinoma risk in a dose-dependent manner: population-based and in vitro studies.* Gut, (2012).

[40] Noto, H, et al. *Cancer risk in diabetic patients treated with metformin: a systematic review and meta-analysis.* PLoS One, (2012). , e33411.

[41] Jin, F, et al. *Evaluation of the association studies of single nucleotide polymorphisms and hepatocellular carcinoma: a systematic review.* J Cancer Res Clin Oncol, (2011). , 1095-1104.

[42] Tian, C, et al. *Variant in PNPLA3 is associated with alcoholic liver disease.* Nat Genet, (2010). , 21-23.

[43] Sookoian, S, & Pirola, C. J. *Meta-analysis of the influence of I148M variant of patatin-like phospholipase domain containing 3 gene (PNPLA3) on the susceptibility and histological severity of nonalcoholic fatty liver disease.* Hepatology, (2011). , 1883-1894.

[44] Valenti, L, & Fargion, S. *Patatin-like phospholipase domain containing-3 Ile148Met and fibrosis progression after liver transplantation.* Hepatology, (2011). , 1484.

[45] Guyot, E, et al. *PNPLA3 rs738409, hepatocellular carcinoma occurrence and risk model prediction in patients with cirrhosis.* J Hepatol, (2012).

Chapter 2

Contrast-Enhanced Ultrasonography (CEUS) of Liver Masses — Principles, Clinical Applications, Drawbacks

R. Badea and Simona Ioanițescu

Additional information is available at the end of the chapter

http://dx.doi.org/10.5772/55500

1. Introduction

Ultrasonography (US) is one of the most widely used imaging procedures. The main advantages of this investigation over others include it being non-invasive and safe, with no radiation exposure. In addition, its images are provided in "real time", delivering dynamic images with both anatomical and functional information. The images acquired by ultrasonography are sectional and easy to understand. The method is accurate, without distortion. The major disadvantage of ultrasonography is that it is operator dependent, requiring a large number of examinations performed personally in order to reach a high level of proficiency [1]. Additional issues include poorer performance if gas, adipose tissue or bony structures come between the transducer and the region of interest. A number of artifacts, such as reverberations and false reflections, may interfere with the acquisition of the ultrasound image, and need to be recognized and avoided.

Ultrasonography is practiced on a daily basis, both by physicians and specialized personal. Now it is widely accepted that a good correlation of the ultrasonographic data with clinical information is necessary in order to achieve an optimal performance [2]. The proposal that access to US should become generalized and be practiced by every physician within their specialty as a way of completing the clinical examination is increasingly voiced [3]. Liver ultrasonography has been recognized for a long time as an application of US efficient in detecting diffuse liver conditions, hepatic tumors, vascular abnormalities, post-traumatic lesions as well as in guiding interventional procedures [4, 5, 6, 7, 8, 9].

Ultrasonography is a multimodal examination, meaning that the final report and basis for the diagnosis, is a complex one, obtained through multiple procedures. Each procedure brings specific data in relation to the underlying principle of operation. The main US component is bidimensional ultrasonography ("grey scale" ultrasound). It consists of sectional images, presented on a grey scale, with each shade of grey representing a density (in fact, an acoustic impedance). "Grey scale" ultrasonography is a dynamic examination that allows the overall evaluation of the liver, with measurements of the hepatic lobes, identification of liver segments, as well as characterization of texture and echogenicity (in relation with the degree of fat infiltration and fibrosis). Grey scale US also enables the detection and evaluation of normal anatomical structures (bile ducts, vessels) and of pathological elements (mainly liver masses). Elastography, an additional component, realizes a quantitative and qualitative (using color coding) characterization of the elasticity of the liver parenchyma [10, 11, 12]. The Doppler procedure represents the basis for evaluating the flow within liver vessels. There is also the spectral version of this application which provides quantitative data (direction of flow, flow velocities, debits, etc) and a color coded version that gives information regarding the presence and the direction of blood flow in the region of interest [13, 14]. Ultrasonography using intravenous (i.v.) contrast agents (CEUS) is a procedure that observes the blood flow in a reference region by revealing the harmonic echoes [15]. Recently, a number of other applications have been developed, many of them based on the mathematical processing of the image. These are meant to optimize the information, enabling quantification, for example, and even allow an automatization of the US diagnosis [16]. Generally speaking, ultrasonography is often the first imaging exploration performed after the clinical exam. As a method, it has proven its value in many respects, including in the detection of liver tumors. In its standard form, however, it is not sensitive enough to characterize and establish the nature of these lesions, despite the many technical advances that have been made [17].

2. The principles and physics of contrast enhanced ultrasonography

The use of contrast in ultrasonography represents a huge advance for this investigation. Even though Doppler ultrasound has a certified role and is the recognized technique for detecting vascular abnormalities in large vessels, it is only after the introduction of contrast agents that we can talk about an exact and reproducible evaluation of microcirculation with the help of ultrasound.

Contrast enhanced ultrasonography (CEUS) consists of injecting gas 'microbubbles' into the systemic circulation. The contrast agent (CA) used is made of small bubbles close in size to red blood cell. These microbubbles contain low soluble gases encapsulated into a biocompatible membrane which may have variable composition – lipids, proteins or biopolymers. The membrane can be either rigid or flexible with a thickness between10-200 nm [18]. Basically, like in any other contrast based imaging procedure, the CEUS exam consists of a "bolus" administration of the contrast media through a superficial peripheral vein. Due to their extremely small size, the microbubbles pass through the pulmonary circulation and then disseminate into the systemic circulation through the arterial blood stream. The contrast agent remains in the blood stream for about 4-5 minutes. There is also a parenchymal phase at the level of the liver and spleen because the contrast agent is captured by the reticuloendothelial system and/or it becomes adherent to the hepatic sinusoids [19]. Unlike the contrast agents used for CT or MRI, the gas used for CEUS is eliminated through the air-ways 10-15 minutes after administration, while the substances that make up the membrane are eliminated through the kidney or metabolized by the liver. The contrast media used in ultrasonography have no toxicity and the technique is less harmful to patients when compared with other investigations.

The contrast enhanced examination is based on the emission of harmonic echoes by the CA when this passes through an ultrasound beam that has a mechanical index of 0.09 – 0.11. The mechanical index (MI) represents a value that is directly correlated with the biological effect of the ultrasounds upon the tissues. This index is variable depending on the ultrasound machine, but it is basically conditioned by the acoustic power of the ultrasounds beam. The acoustic power (AP), measured in Pascals, represents the energy of the sound beam acting on a target, for example a group of red cells or the contrast agent inside the blood stream. Usually, at high values of the AP, up to MegaPa, the micro bubbles are "broken" and an irregular, non-linear signal is generated. At low values of the AP (30-70 kPa) the microbubbles vibrate in a particular, non-linear manner, producing alternating contractions and relaxations, thus generating harmonic echoes.

The ultrasound equipment produces a separation of the harmonic echoes generated by the CA within the blood stream from the echoes generated by the surrounding tissues. This separation may be realized by modulating the phase and the amplitude of the US beam. There are multiple US generating techniques within the transducer that generate harmonic echoes within the CA. Techniques of pulse inversion ("Pulse Inversion", "Power Pulse Inversion", "Cadence Contrast Pulse Sequencing") perform a "subtraction" of the tissue echoes by alternative emission of pulses found in an inversed phase. A "Vascular Recognition Imaging" technique introduces the Doppler principle in the analysis of the returned signals, allowing a color coding of the red cells in relation to their direction of flow.

Practically, CEUS consists of an injection of a contrast agent, prepared at the time of use, into a cubital vein. This is followed by a bolus of 10 cc saline solution. The region of interest, previously identified during the "grey scale" exam, is continuously observed on the monitor. The monitor may be divided into two identical, real-time images, one using fundamental, "grey scale", echoes and the other one using harmonic echoes obtained by exposure to a sound beam with a low mechanical index (0.09 – 0.11). The examination continues for 90 seconds. After this time the exploration may be intermittent. CEUS is focused on a single region of interest, usually a mass. The exploration of another mass requires either a "breaking" of the bubbles inside the mass, performed with special software or using the CFM technique, or a repetition of the CEUS exam after another contrast administration focused on the second lesion. There are no risks for the patient, so the injection of the CA can be repeated as often as needed.

Using CEUS in the exploration of the liver has special features that arise from the double vascularity of this organ – through the portal vein (two thirds) and through the arterial system (one third). The sequence of blood entering the liver is first arterial (up to 30 seconds) and then portal (30 to 90 seconds, with little variation). This vascular discrimination (similar to the one obtained by contrast CT or MRI) allows for gathering information regarding the circulatory bed (types of feeding vessels, tumor circulatory volume) of a tumor. The presence of arterio-venous communications is characteristic for the neoplastic circulation and in CEUS is expressed by the "wash-out" process. This phenomenon begins at the end of the arterial phase and/or during the venous phase, is persistent and is characteristic for neoplastic processes in 90 % of cases [20]. There are studies that correlate the wash-out speed of the tumor with its aggressiveness, attributing CEUS a prognostic value.

An important component of the CEUS exam is represented by the quantitative analysis of the data. This consists of a representation in time of the acoustic impedance variation in one or more predetermined regions of interest. A graphic is obtained that can be correlated with hemodynamic parameters, like the time of maximum systolic ascent in the region of interest, the volume of the circulatory bed, presence and scale of the arteriovenous shunts, etc. All these elements are indicators for the quality of a specific circulatory bed [21].

The advantages of the CEUS technique are summarized in Table 1 and include the lack of ionizing radiation exposure, the non invasive character of the method, as well as very good spatial and temporal resolution [22]. The method is safe for patients, with very few cases of anaphylaxis having been reported (about 0.001% of the total number of investigations). It is therefore recommended in some centres as the firstline procedure for assessment of liver nodules. Contrast CT not only exposes the patient to ionizing radiation, but iodine based contrast agents can be toxic and produce allergic reactions. CT scan imaging may also be less sensitive, "losing" or failing to capture the early arterial phase in highly vascular tumors.

• very good spatial resolution;
• high temporal resolution – it is a "real time" examination;
• it reveals very slow blood flow or stagnant blood streams;
• non-ionizing examination;
• lack of anaphylaxis;
• the contrast agent is eliminated through the air-ways;
• can be repeated as often as needed

Table 1. Advantages of the CEUS examination

It should also be recognized that CEUS exploration has a number of limitations, as summarized in Table 2. It is dependent on expensive and sophisticated equipment that raises the cost of the investigation. The harmonic image is depending on good quality 2D image. Deeper lesions are harder to visualize and attenuation may represent a limit in detecting tumors located further from the transducer. Last, but not least the investigation is operator dependent and often the information that is obtained must be correlated with the clinical data and biochemical functional information.

• expensive and sophisticated equipment;
• high cost of the exploration compared with the standard investigation;
• operator dependent;
• it depends on a good quality 2D image;
• low quality information in case of attenuation like in liver steatosis;
• it investigates a single region of interest;

Table 2. Limitations of CEUS examination

3. CEUS and the assessment of benign liver tumors

The imaging/ultrasonographic contribution to the detection of benign liver tumors is not insignificant. Benign lesions are numerous, affecting about 20% of the population [23]. They are frequently detected following ultrasonography, which is widely available and represents a common investigation in any abdominal complaint. CEUS exploration can distinguish between benign and malignant tumors and consequently can halt the diagnostic algorithm when a mass detected by 2D ultrasonography is characterized by CEUS as being benign. In this way the numbers of investigations is optimal and the patient's discomfort is significantly reduced. There a multiple benign liver masses, however, and not all of them have CEUS characteristic features. Their ultrasonographic aspect is often similar and their discrimination may require additional criteria [24]. Among the lesions that present specific circulation patterns which can be defined when analyzed by CEUS are cysts, hemangiomas, adenoma and benign focal hyperplasia (table 3).

Tumor	Arterial phase	Portal phase	Delayed phase	2D feature
Cyst	No uptake	No uptake	No uptake	Transsonic
Hemangioma	"Ring-like" peripheral uptake	Centripetal enhancement resembling "buds"	Complete uptake	Hyperechoic Well-defined Compressibility "Mirror" effect
Focal nodular hyperplasia	Central enhancement with a "spoked wheel" distribution of the CA	Complete enhancement with an isoechoic appearance compared with liver parenchyma	Isoechoic aspect when compared with the liver parenchyma	Echoic scar in the centre of the lesion Arterial signal in the centre of the tumor
Adenoma	Inhomogeneous uptake	Discrete wash-out Iso or hypoechoic aspect compared to liver parenchyma	Discrete wash-out, Iso or hypoechoic aspect compared to liver parenchyma	Hypoechoic nodule Non-cirrhotic liver

(*) The information presented in the table is referring to typical situations. In practice, there are variations of the 2D or CEUS aspects that require further investigations

Table 3. CEUS and 2D ultrasonographic features in cases of benign liver lesions. (*)

Liver hemangioma. It is the most frequently encountered benign tumor of the liver. It is most often found in women and has a prevalence of about 0.4 – 7.4 % in the population [25]. The mass consists of a vascular, capillary or venous, bundle, rich in fibrotic bands and with no capsule. It may be frequently associated with other benign tumors like cysts or adenomas. Hemangiomas are usually asymptomatic (in very rare cases, when extremely large they may cause a distension of the liver capsule and thrombocytopenia) and have a slow, self-limiting development. In most cases there is just one lesion, but there is also a multicentric type. The grey scale US appearance of hemangiomas is fairly characteristic: a well circumscribed, hyperechoic liver mass, with a slightly hypoechoic centre or periphery (figure 1).

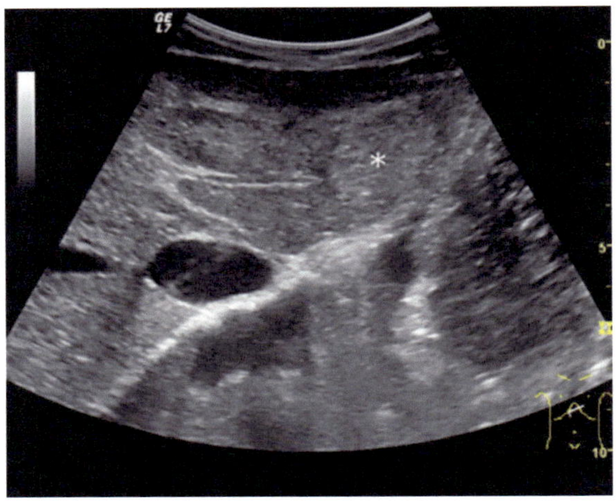

Figure 1. Liver hemangioma. The lesion is found within the left lobe (asterisk) and has a characteristic appearance on "grey scale" ultrasound: well circumscribed, hypoechoic nodule with irregular margins.

Hemangiomas do not cause vascular or biliary ducts invasion. But they may produce an effect of posterior acoustic enhancement. On closer inspection the operator can observe this effect by changing the aspect of the transducer in combination with profound compression. When the hemangioma is located in contact with the diaphragm it can generate a "mirror" effect that leads to a reproduction of the image in the lung parenchyma. Hemangiomas do not usually show signal on the Doppler investigation as flow velocities inside them are very low. Additionally, in many cases intratumoral ischemia or fibrotic scars will develop. Often, the ultrasonographic diagnostic criteria are clear enough and in most situations the conventional ultrasound which first detects the nodule, is sufficient to characterize the lesion. But there are circumstances when 2D ultrasound is not sufficient for tumor characterization and thus CEUS is needed. In the presence of severe steatosis as well as in patients undergoing chemotherapy for various neoplastic conditions, the appearance of a hemangioma may alter and become "atypical". Also in patients with liver cirrhosis, a hemangioma may be misinterpreted for a hepatocellular carcinoma or a large regeneration nodule. Extremely large hemangiomas may have a heterogeneous structure due to possible hemorrhage or ischemia developed inside the lesion, which can alter their appearance. Last but not least, CEUS can be very useful in reassuring both operator and patient that a nodule accidentally found during an ultrasound exam is benign.

http://dx.doi.org/10.5772/55500

The appearance of a hemangioma on CEUS is characterized by a peripheral, ring-like, clear enhancement during the arterial phase (figure 2a). This process is continuous and slow and is followed the appearance of contrast "buds" inwardly oriented (figure 2b). In the end, after several minutes of observation, a complete enhancement of the hemangioma is observed (figure 2c). Therefore a pattern of progressive and centripetal enhancement of a nodule is the characteristic feature for the diagnosis of hemangioma [26].

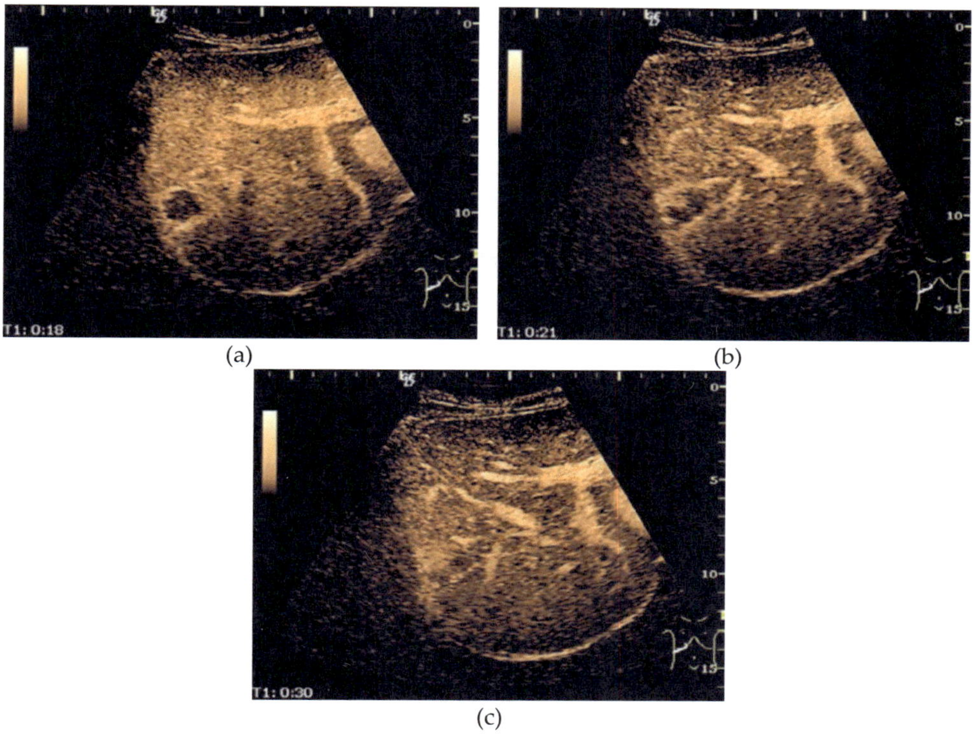

Figure 2. Liver hemangioma. a. CEUS performed during the arterial phase (18 seconds since contrast media injection) shows a well defined "ring" around the nodule. b. The appearance of the contrast "buds" suggests the centripetal character of CA progression. c. At the end of the arterial phase there is complete enhancement of the lesion with contrast agent.

The uptake may take variable amounts of time, from tens of seconds to several minutes (even tens of minutes), depending on the size of the lesion and the type of circulatory bed (figure 3a; figure 3b; figure 3c).

A particular type of hemangioma is the arterialized type. It is characterized by accelerated, complete uptake during the arterial phase. It corresponds to circulatory alterations characterized by an important arterial flow. In this situations a differential diagnosis with hypervascular metastases or HCC is difficult and thus a correlation with other imaging techniques is mandatory [27].

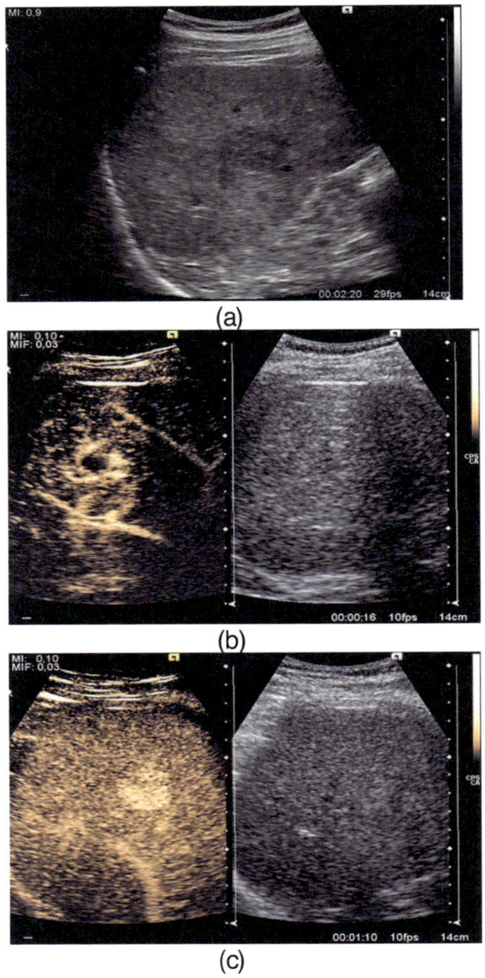

Figure 3. a. "Atypical" liver hemangioma. This is the case of a female patient undergoing chemotherapy for breast cancer. There is increased echogenicity of the liver suggesting therapy induced dystrophy. In the middle of the right lobe there is a hypoechoic, solid lesion that raises the possibility of a liver metastasis. b. CEUS exam shows a "ring" enhancement of the lesion during the arterial phase (16th second). c. CEUS exam reveals a complete enhancement of the nodule at the end of the portal phase (70th second). The enhancement process was centripetal (from periphery towards the centre). The diagnosis is certainly of hemangioma. The case demonstrates the role of the CEUS in patients undergoing oncologic treatments who present liver nodules.

Liver cysts. Liver cysts are serous collection circumscribed by cuboidal epithelium. They are frequently encountered during 2D ultrasound, especially in women. Usually they measure less than 20 mm and can present as single or multiple lesions. An involvement of the entire liver is rare. The grey scale US aspect of cysts is that of a well defined, transsonic lesion with posterior acoustic enhancement. The walls of a cyst are very thin and often difficult to distinguish. Inside the cyst there may be thin septa and sometimes deposits. Cysts show no signal on the CFM (color flow mode) interrogation. A hydatid cyst additionally presents

http://dx.doi.org/10.5772/55500

daughter cysts and abundant deposits inside. The size of a hydatid cyst is usually larger and the 2D pattern may present in one of several ways, including organization as a solid mass. In such cases the differential diagnosis includes a malignant tumor. In addition to these cases, a CEUS examination is indicated in cases of hypoechoic cysts identified in patients with liver steatosis or cirrhosis, when identifying a vascular signal inside the lesion is determinant in establishing the differential diagnosis (figure 4a; figure 4b). During the arterial phase cysts are highlighted even at sizes of 2 mm, due to their transsonic appearance that contrasts the arterialized surrounding parenchyma.

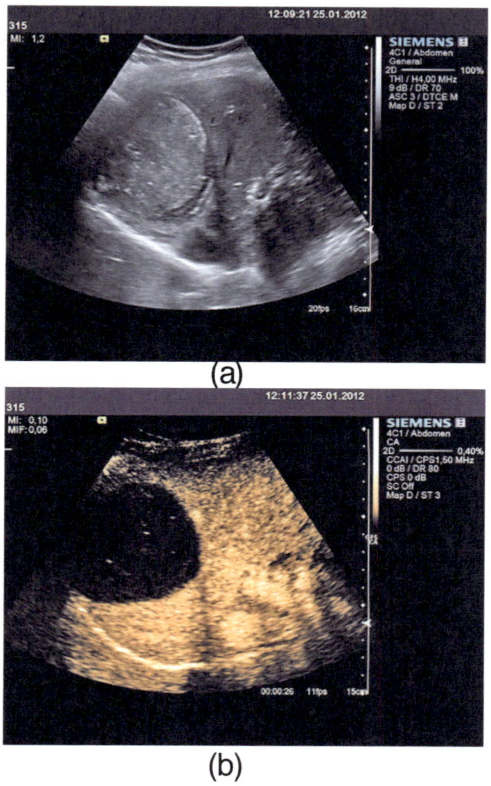

Figure 4. a. Inactive, solid, organized hydatid cyst of the liver (Gharbi classification, 1981). b. Organized hydatid cyst. CEUS exam demonstrates the lack of vascularity within the tumor and thus contributes to the decisive exclusion of a malignant liver tumor.

Focal nodular hyperplasia (FNH). FNH is a pseudotumor characterized by an area of normal liver cells proliferated around an arterialized scar. Focal nodular hyperplasia has an abundant portal circulatory bed. It is more frequent in women and its development may be linked with the use of oral contraceptives [28]. There is no risk of malignant transformation or spontaneous rupture. The lesion may be unique or there can be multiple lesions. The grey scale ultrasonographic aspect is that of a solid lesion with no capsule of its own (figure 5).

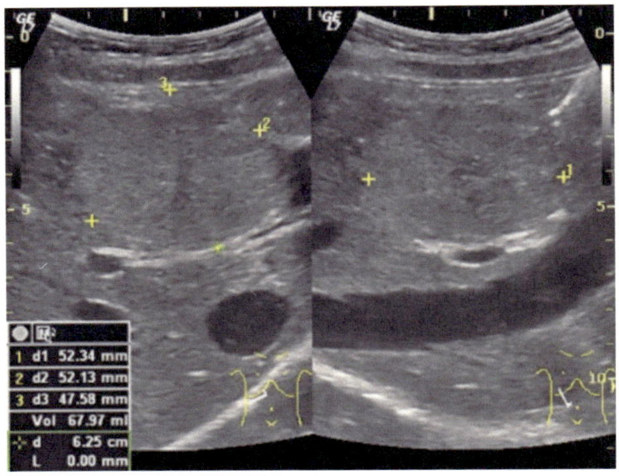

Figure 5. Focal nodular hyperplasia. "Grey scale" ultrasound examination. Perpendicular view through the left lobe. The lesion is solid and well-defined. In the centre of the lesion there is a linear structure that belongs to the typical, central scar (asterisk).

The central scar is more obvious in larger lesions and it presents as a linear, echoic structure. The CFM examination reveals a vascular signal in this area, while pulsed Doppler ultrasound detects arterial flow (figure 6a; figure 6b).

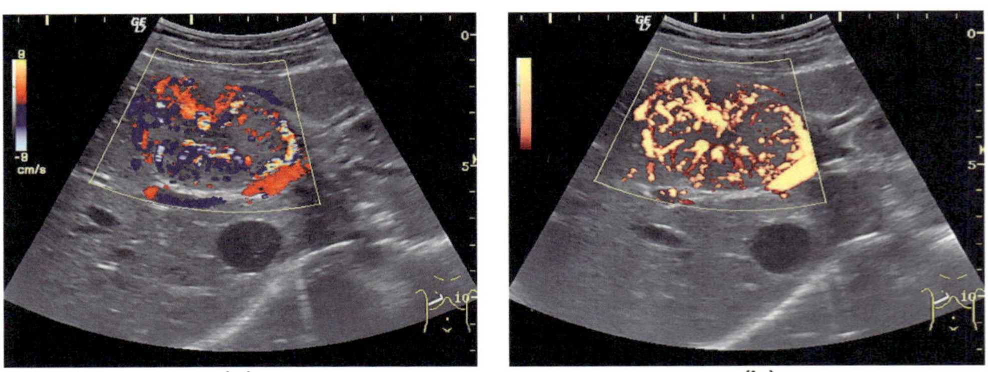

(a) (b)

Figure 6. Focal nodular hyperplasia. a. CFM examination. The lesion has a high vascular signal. The vessels have "spoked wheel" spatial distribution. b. "Power mode" exam. "Spoked wheel" vascular pattern.

The CEUS behavior of FNH is characterized by an accelerated uptake in the centre of the lesion during the arterial phase, with a radial distribution, creating a "spoked wheel" appearance (figure 7a). The use of image post-processing procedures allows the identification of the vessels that make up the lesion, as well as their spatial distribution (figure 7b).

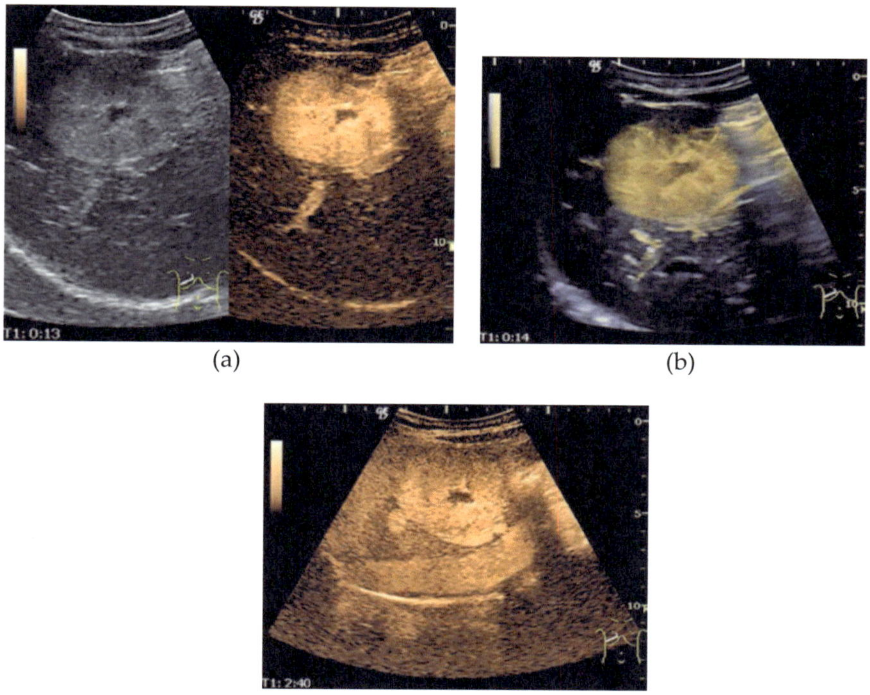

(a) (b) (c)

Figure 7. a. Focal nodular hyperplasia. CEUS exam during arterial phase. In the 13th second after contrast administration there is complete enhancement of the lesion. In the centre of the lesion there is a hypoechoic structure (the tumoral scar). The tumor pedicle can also be visualized. b. Focal nodular hyperplasia. Combined CEUS examination, using image post-processing techniques, that allows visualization of the spatial distribution of the vessels, which present a radiant orientation. c. Focal nodular hyperplasia (same case as figures 5, 6a, 6b). The CEUS examination performed after 160 seconds from contrast media injection reveals a similar aspect of the lesion. There is no contrast wash-out, thus excluding malignancy.

Liver adenoma. A liver adenoma is an accumulation of hepatic cells, with no biliary structures or Kupffer cells. Its development can be induced by the use of oral contraceptives. Adenomas may also arise in patients with metabolic diseases such as type I glycogen storage disease, as well as in long term administration of anabolic androgenic hormones. Adenomas are arterialized but they do not contain portal vessels. They may be very large in size and thus become symptomatic through pain and intratumoral bleeding. In 5% of the cases adenomas may undergo malignant transformation [30]. Risk of malignant transformation as well as the risk of rupture within the peritoneal cavity can make detected and characterized adenomas indications for surgery. The grey scale ultrasound aspect is that of a well-circumscribed, hypoechoic, solid tumor. The vascular signal evaluated by CFM is non characteristic. After contrast media administration, during the arterial phase there is an irregular enhancement (due to intratumoral bleeding) (figure 8a,figure 8b). During the portal venous phase there is moderate wash-out which makes the tumor look iso or hypoechoic compared with the surrounding liver parenchyma. This behavior is seen in the delayed phase as well. The slow wash-out, the hypoechoic aspect during the portal and delayed phases as well as the moderate and inhomogeneous uptake in the arterial phase are elements that may cause misinterpretation of adenomas for malignant tumors.

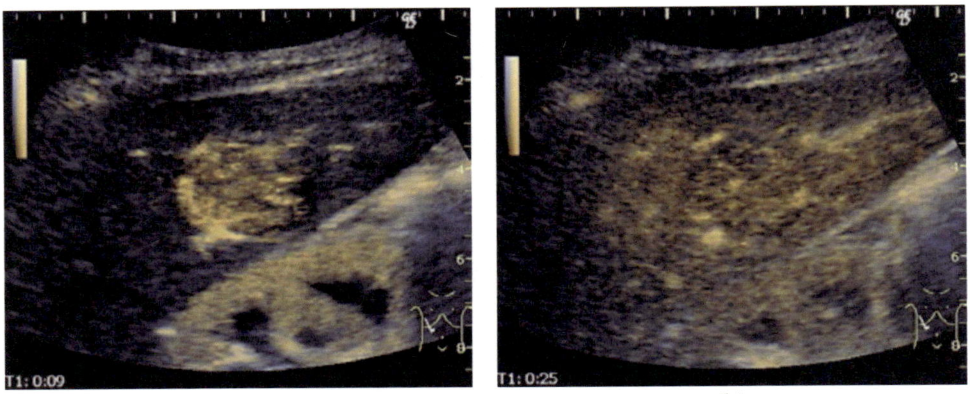

(a) (b)

Figure 8. Liver adenoma, CEUS examination. a. during the arterial phase the tumor presents inhomogeneous uptake. b. CEUS shows moderate contrast wash-out at the end of the arterial phase.

The discrimination of adenomas from HCC is often based on the appearance of the liver on which it developed being normal or dystrophic. As HCC can arise in the absence of chronic liver disease, if there is any cause for doubt additional imaging techniques and/or liver biopsy should be considered. Similarly, distinguishing an adenoma from a metastasis is difficult and the lesion may need additional investigation to complete the diagnosis.

4. CEUS and the assessment of malignant liver tumors

Malignant tumors of the liver represent the main application of ultrasonography. The method can detect these masses within an evocative clinical context (a typical example is that of an oncologic patient who presents with liver nodules or that of a patient with cirrhosis that during follow-up develops a liver nodule) or by chance, during a routine ultrasound examination. The spatial resolution of ultrasonography is sufficient to allow the detection of nodules as small as 10 mm (table 4).

The CEUS examination has a high, but not absolute, specificity! The method contributes to the consolidation of the clinical and grey scale ultrasonographic diagnosis of malignant tumor. The final diagnosis (tumor characterization) is based on an accumulation of criteria, among which is the character of the liver on which a nodule develops (cirrhotic or non-cirrhotic liver), the clinical presentation and the biochemical and functional data of the patient. The intensity of intratumoral echogenicity as the CA crosses the nodule is compared with that of the neighboring liver parenchyma during the same vascular phase.

Tumor	Arterial phase	Portal venous phase	Delayed phase	"Grey scale" ultrasound (2D)
Hepatocellular carcinoma	Intense enhancement Hyperechoic aspect	Moderate/Intense wash-out Hypoechoic or isoechoic aspect	Moderate/Intense wash-out Hypoechoic aspect	Solid tumor Inhomogeneous structure "Basket-like" appearance of the CFM vascular pattern Arterialized circulation Portal invasion
Cholangiocarcinoma	Moderate, inhomogeneous uptake Hyperechoic / Isoechoic aspect	Moderate wash-out Hypoechoic aspect	Moderate or intense wash-out Hypoechic aspect	Solid tumor located in the hilum or subcapsulary Bile ducts dilations oriented towards the tumor
Hypovascular metastases	Peripheral uptake Hypoechoic aspect	Peripheral wash-out Hypoechoic aspect	Intense wash-out Hypoechoic aspect	Multiple, solid masses Involvement of all liver lobes
Hypervascular metastases	Intense uptake Hyperechoic aspect	Moderate wash-out Hypoechoic aspect	Intense wash-out Hypoechoic aspect	

Table 4. CEUS and 2D ultrasonographic features of malignant liver masses

5. Hepatocellular Carcinoma (HCC)

Hepatocellular carcinoma is the most frequent primary tumor of the liver [31]. In the vast majority of the cases (over 80%) HCC develops on a liver already affected by cirrhosis. Liver cirrhosis is defined in morphological terms as a process of fibrosis and reorganization. The reorganization of the liver parenchyma leads to the development of variable size, even millimetric, nodules with an ubiquitous distribution involving the entire liver and representing the origin of hepatocellular carcinoma. HCC develops from one or more cirrhosis nodules. Many prospective and retrospective studies have demonstrated this continuity. The development of high resolution imaging techniques that can reliably distinguish between regenerative and cancerous nodules necessitates the accomplishment of practical systematic and validated approaches for their clinically relevant application. In addition to a role in the characterization of such nodules in the diagnosis of cancer, some US characteristics are thought to identify individuals at high risk of developing a cancer. The ultrasonographic pattern of a "restless liver", for example, is recognized as a "risk" model for the development of hepatocellular carcinoma [32].

The work group of the World Gastroenterology Congress in 1994 agreed upon an anatomical and clinical systematization of the nodules that considers both the presence of the nodules (at the moment of their imaging detection) as well as the dynamics of their development. Regeneration nodules, low dysplastic nodules, high dysplastic nodules with outbreaks of hepatocelllular carcinoma, incipient hepatocellular carcinoma (< 2 cm) and typical hepatocarcinoma can be identified in the cirrhotic liver [33]. This systematization also considers the existence of a vascular dynamics inside the nodules which is considered a key element of carcinogenesis [34, 35]. Inside the dysplastic nodules there is a progressive reduction – until disappearance – of the portal vessels and a proportional growth of the arterial vessels during the multiplication process of the neoplastic cells. The tumoral circulatory bed is made of arterial vessels with a disorganized, chaotic spatial distribution, arteriovenous shunts and the precapillary sphincter of the arterioles is missing. The vascular characteristics of the neoplastic nodules are considered to be determinant for their echogenicity in contrast with that of the surrounding liver parenchyma. In conclusion, high dysplastic nodules are usually hypoechoic, while incipient nodules of highly differentiated hepatocellular carcinoma are usually isoechoic [36].

The Liver Cancer Study Group of Japan defined the following types of nodules:

a. a small nodule with ill defined margins, size under 20 mm, consisting of well differentiated cells and portal vessels (about 85% of the cases). It may contain areas of low differentiated cells with a different potential of multiplication, realizing a "nodule in nodule" pattern;

b. a small nodule with ill defined margins, round shape and non-tumoral capsule. In most situations it is made of well differentiated cells (about 75%) and sometimes (about 20% of cases) it may present histological signs of portal invasion;

c. a tumor nodule with extratumoral buds consisting in most cases of low differentiated cells;

d. a multinodular pattern made of several nodules in contact with each other, realizing an irregular delineation. They consist of moderate or low differentiated cells;

e. an infiltrative pattern characterized by a vague, irregular delineation. In most situations it is made of low differentiated cells and/or transitional hepatocytes and cholangiocytes, generating a mixed tumor between the two cellular types.

On the "grey scale" ultrasound exploration a 10 – 20 mm incipient HCC has the aspect of a heterogenous nodule with hypoechoic and hyperechoic areas inside, an appearance that is influenced by the fat content and the degree of cellular differentiation [37]. The Doppler exploration shows a continuous, portal vascular signal oriented towards the tumor [38]. The undulating character of the flow draws attention to a more significant arterial component, which often correlates with poorly differentiated tumors.

The advanced form of HCC may have the following characteristics: demarcation by a halo and lateral shadow (produced by the fibrous capsule of the tumor); inhomogeneous structure (generated by fibrotic and vascular bands which alternate with areas of intact and necrotic tumoral tissue); irregular, ill defined margins (suggesting an invasion of the surrounding liver parenchyma and of the portal vascular bed); posterior acoustic shadowing (generated by the softer consistency of the tumor compared with the normal liver parenchyma). The distinctive vascular aspect, obtained by using the color coded technique of the blood flow (CFM), is that of a basket pattern, characterized by the presence of arterial vessels that circumscribe the tumor and feed it from outside [39]. The spectral exploration demonstrates accelerated flow velocities and altered impedance indexes, since the vascular resistance of the circulatory bed is lower in the absence of precapillary sphincters. On CEUS the aspect of the HCC is typical and is the consequence of its vascular features described earlier (Figure 9). It is characterized by accelerated uptake during the arterial phase, contrast wash-out during the portal venous phase and a hypoechoic appearance in the delayed phase. The wash-out speed is conditioned by the degree of cellular differentiation of the tumor, the lower the differentiation the faster the wash-out (figure 10a; figure 10b;).

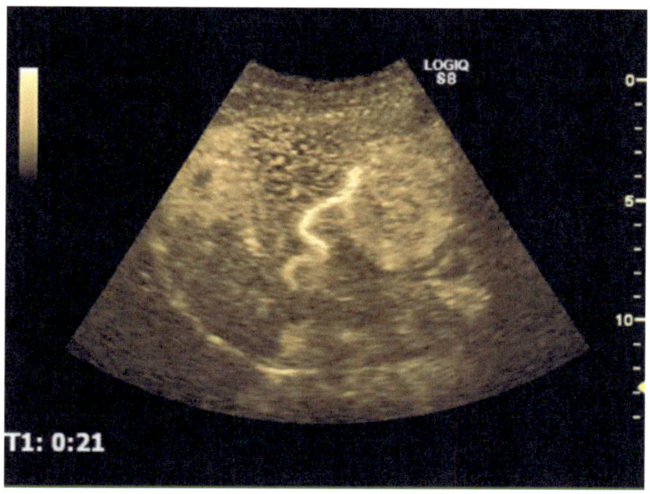

Figure 9. Multicentric, large hepatocellular carcinoma. Two large lesions are visualized during the arterial phase. One of the lesions presents an important feeding artery.

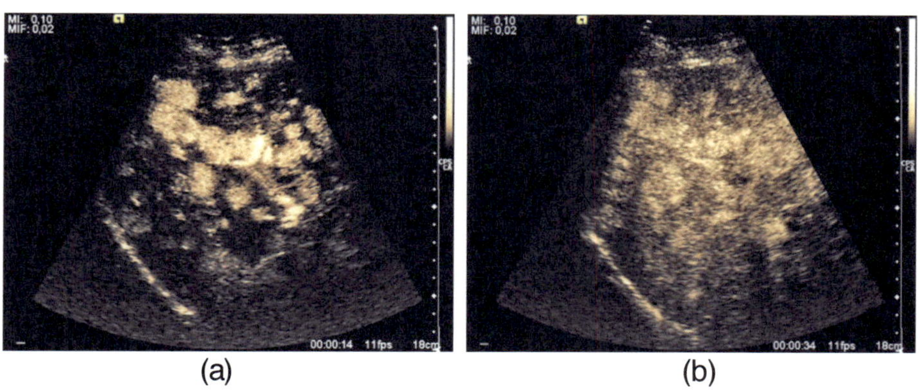

Figure 10. Multicentric, large hepatocellular carcinoma. a. CEUS examination (arterial phase) demonstrates the presence of highly enhancing, numerous nodules. b. The hypoechoic appearance of the lesions can be visualized (34th second), suggesting their malignant nature and the low differentiating grade of the tumor.

The exploration allows the discrimination of a malignant invasion of the portal vein from thrombosis based on the behavior during the arterial phase: in case of tumor invasion, the signal is simultaneous with the one inside the hepatic artery, while during the portal phase it loses its signal and becomes obvious (Figure 11) [40].

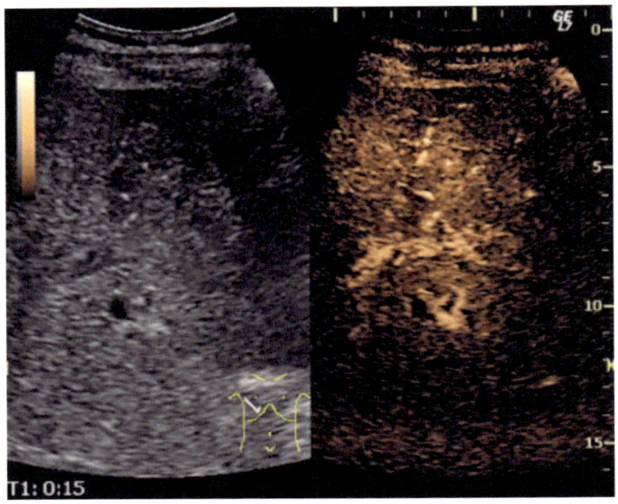

Figure 11. Tumor invasion of the portal vein. Dual harmonics examination with i.v. contrast, that shows a filling with echoes of the right portal vein on the left and contrast media uptake within the portal lumen during the arterial phase (15th second).

6. CEUS assessment of cholangiocarcinoma (CCC)

Cholangiocarcinoma is a rare primary malignancy (3 – 7 % of all malignant liver tumors) which usually develops in a histologically normal liver [41]. There are conditions, however, that present higher risks for developing CCC. These included primary sclerosing cholangitis, choledochal cysts, Caroli disease or intrahepatic biliary lithiasis [30]. The origin of CCC is in the small biliary ducts and tumour development is frequently associated with an early appearance of jaundice. The tumor may present a nodular pattern (most cases), an intraductal circumscribed pattern, or a periductal infiltrative type. The nodular type is well-circumscribed, with a fibrotic structure and moderate or poorly differentiated cells. It is frequently associated with metastases in the surrounding parenchyma (developed by contiguity as well as through portal veins) as well as lymph nodes in the hepatic hilum [42]. On the grey scale ultrasound examination, an early CCC is undetectable. In this situation the diagnosis is based on indirect signs, the main one being the dilatation of the intrahepatic bile ducts. Biochemical serum tests, especially those elevated and reflecting abnormal biliary function such as CA 19 – 9 and CEA, may be useful for diagnosis [28]. When the tumor is advanced stage the diagnosis is based on the presence of a solid mass, well delineated, but without a capsule, adjacent to the bile ducts

http://dx.doi.org/10.5772/55500

(often in the hilum). The bile ducts may be well dilated. The vascular signal detected upon CFM exploration is weaker than that detected in HCC. The vessels are arterial and have a chaotic spatial distribution. The tumor may be unique or multicentric and it may have a subcapsular localization. An indirect element that sustains the diagnosis is the development of the tumor in a normal liver. The CEUS exam may present an inhomogeneous uptake during the arterial phase, the behavior being uncharacteristic. During the portal venous phase the appearance is hypoechoic and it persists this way in the delayed phase [43].

7. CEUS in the assessment of liver metastases

The liver represents the second site for malignant secondary tumors in oncology. There are usually multiple lesions and rarely single. The common sites of origin are mainly represented by the digestive tract, lungs, breast and pancreatic head [44]. They have fewer vessels than primary malignancies of the liver. During their evolution they may develop hemorrhage, areas of ischemia and necrosis, as well as areas of fibrosis and calcifications. These features contribute to imaging appearances that are extremely diverse and uncharacteristic for their origin when assessed by US. In essence, in a patient with a known neoplastic condition, or in the situation of weight loss in the context of a malignancy, the presence of multiple nodules, measuring more than 10 mm, involving the whole liver, is suggestive for the presence of liver metastases. The CFM exploration does not bring significant information. The CEUS exam is based on demonstrating a hypoechoic aspect during the portal venous phase and delayed phase, which is highly suspicious for malignancy. During the arterial phase metastases may present either a hypo or a hypervascular pattern (figure 12; figure 13a, figure 13b).

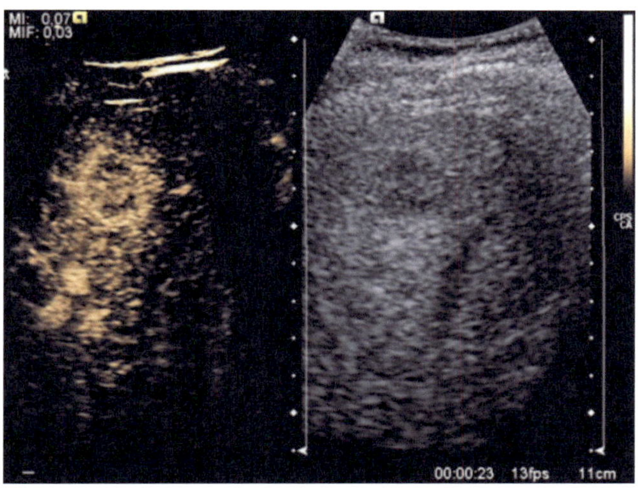

Figure 12. Liver metastasis (breast neoplasm). CEUS exploration shows a vascular mass 23 seconds after contrast media injection.

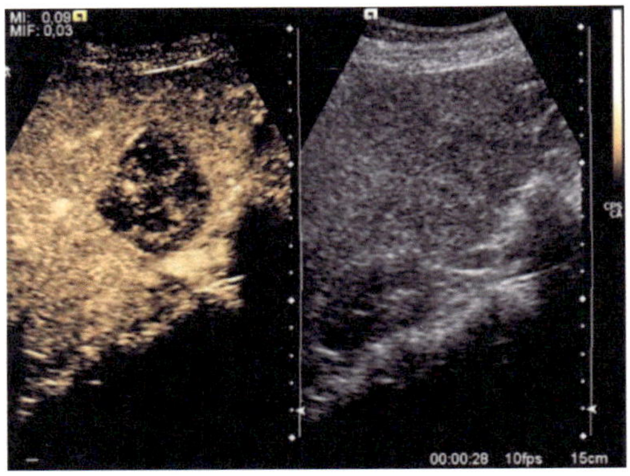

(a)

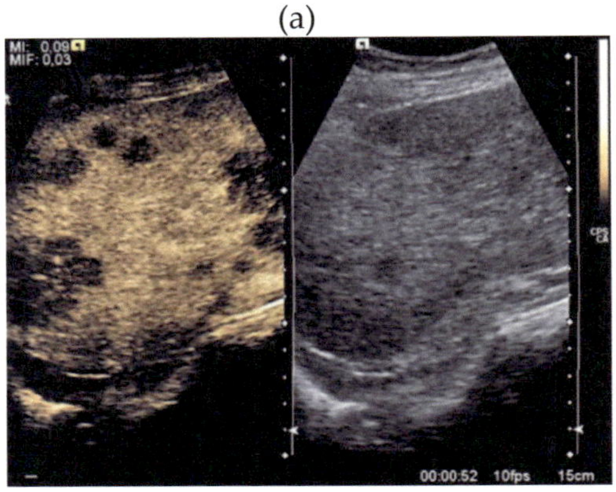

(b)

Figure 13. a. Liver metastasis (colon neoplasm). CEUS examination reveals a hypoechoic mass 28 seconds after injection. b. Liver metastasis (colon neoplasm). CEUS examination shows multiple hypoechoic masses at 52 seconds after injection (portal venous phase). Typical appearance.

Hypervascular mets may be associated to carcinoid tumors, melanomas, sarcomas and thyroid or renal tumors. The role of CEUS in the evaluation of liver metastases is focused on at least two applications: a. detection of metastases smaller than 10 mm and counting them. The method significantly increases the sensitivity of ultrasound and gets it closer to that of i.v. contrast-enhanced CT [45]. b. assessment of therapy efficiency (chemotherapy and chemoembolization). In this regard the method can document the disappearance of the circulatory bed and suggests an efficient treatment.

8. CEUS in the assessment of other types of liver masses

This category includes non neoplastic liver masses that are quiet frequently encountered. Ultrasonography often detects such lesions. The US exam must clarify whether there are evolving features or not and if there are special risks for the patient (table 5).

Liver mass	Arterial phase	Portal venous phase	Delayed phase	"Grey scale" US
Liver abscess	Peripheral uptake and liver parenchyma uptake Hypoechoic/Transsonic aspect	Echoic appearance of the liver parenchyma Hypoechoic aspect	Echoic appearance of the liver parenchyma Hypoechoic aspect	Hypoechoic or transsonic lesion Semifluid content Intratumoral gas
Focal liver steatosis	Simultaneous uptake with the liver parenchyma	Isoechoic aspect	Isoechoic aspect	Hypoechoic area "Shining" appearance of the liver parenchyma
Regeneration nodule	Weak uptake Hypoechoic aspect	Isoechoic aspect	Isoechoic aspect	Solid nodule, d = 10 – 20 mm Inhomogeneous liver

Table 5. CEUS and "grey scale" US criteria for the diagnosis of non neoplastic masses of the liver.

Liver abscess. Liver abscesses may arise in various circumstances: primary abscesses (in immune deficiency cases) or secondary abscesses in postoperative patients, or associated with sepsis, abdominal abscesses, post traumatic conditions, acute angiocholitis or acute pancreatitis etc. The "grey scale" ultrasound aspect is variable in relation to the number and size of the lesions (figure 14). In general it presents itself as a unique, large mass, well circumscribed, but irregular, with a semi-fluid content and with echoic tissue elements and air inside. It can also present as multiple, smaller size lesions, a situation when their texture may mimic liver metastases. The CFM exploration reveals that the vessels are displaced by the mass and that the abscess has no vascular signal inside.

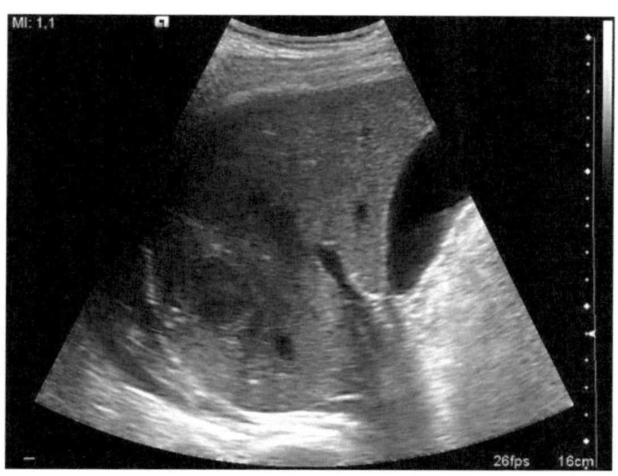

Figure 14. Liver abscess. Hypoechoic mass, with semifluid features, visualized in the right lobe of the liver. There is also right pleural fluid collection.

The CEUS exam shows a progressive uptake in the periphery of the abscess during the arterial phase. This enhancement happens simultaneously with that of the surrounding liver parenchyma which is congested (figure 15a). This aspect is persistent during the portal venous phase as well. During the delayed phase the fluid areas inside the abscess/abscesses are highlighted due to the enhancement of the liver sinusoids and the reticuloendothelial system of the liver (figure 15b) [46].

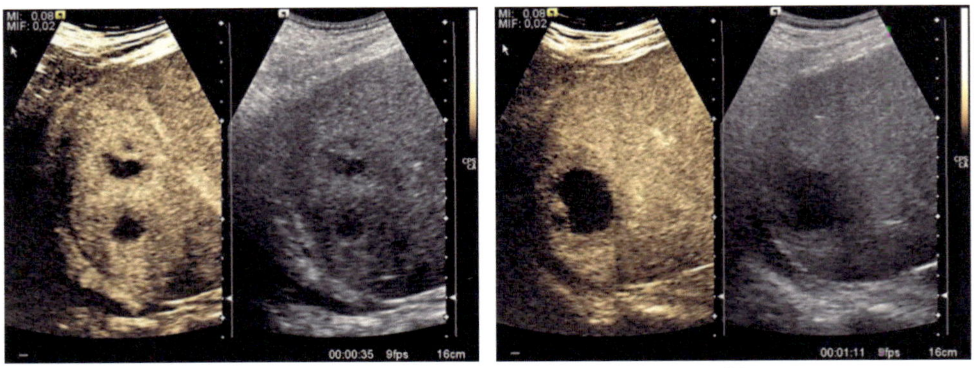

(a) (b)

Figure 15. Liver abscess (same case as figure 14). a. Dual image showing on the left an increased echogenicity of the liver parenchyma during arterial phase. The aspect suggests liver congestion and represents an indirect sign that supports the diagnosis of a liver abscess. b. Portal-venous phase. A decrease of liver echogenicity is noted while the infected collection is emphasized.

Focal liver steatosis. Focal steatosis develops in the context of metabolic conditions, chemotherapy or excessive alcohol consumption. The liver is intensely echoic and presents hypoechoic, rather well circumscribed "islands" or "areas" inside. The Doppler exploration does not reveal additional vessels. The CEUS exam reveals an isoechoic aspect of the liver during the arterial phase. During the portal venous phase and the delayed phase the region of interest is identical with the surrounding liver and thus excludes the presence of a mass.

Regeneration nodules. Regeneration nodules appear as nodular, well circumscribed, hypoechoic masses, usually measuring less than 20 mm. They are often numerous and have a uniform, ubiquitous distribution, involving all the segments of the liver. They may come together as a cluster and form large pseudotumors. This aspect is characteristic for viral liver cirrhosis. These nodules do not present Doppler signals. CEUS exploration is indicated when a certain nodule is larger than the majority of the liver nodules. An increase in size, demonstrated by measurements performed at 6 – 8 weeks, represents an additional indication. Characteristically, the vascular signal is weak or absent during the arterial phase, while in the portal and delayed phases the lesion is persistently isoechoic (figure 16). CEUS is useful in order to exclude an active lesion at the moment of the examination, but it has no prognosis value and that is why the patient must be reexamined at short time intervals [8]. A correlation with the clinical findings and with the values of AFP is mandatory.

http://dx.doi.org/10.5772/55500

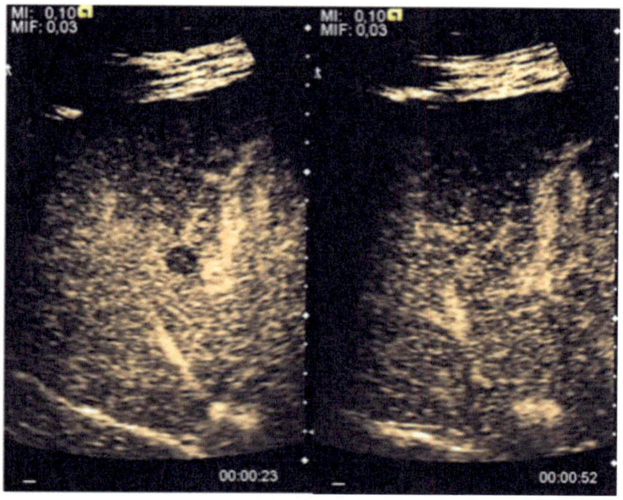

Figure 16. Regeneration nodule. CEUS reveals low irrigation during the arterial phase (23th second) and lack of contrast wash-out during the portal venous phase (52th second).

9. Final remarks

Contrast-enhanced ultrasonography is a noninvasive imaging procedure that allows the gathering of information regarding the dynamics of circulation and the features of the circulatory bed in the region of interest [47]. The investigation is based on the identification of the circulatory phases within the liver – arterial, portal and delayed phase – which are overlapping those identified at contrast CT or MRI. The dynamic analysis of the image in relation with these phases allows the detection and characterization of tumors with similar accuracy to that of CT and MRI [48, 49]. The risks and side effects of the method are insignificant and that is why CEUS must be considered a safe procedure for the patient. This investigation should be commonly used for the characterization of liver nodules developed on liver cirrhosis and suspicion of HCC, regardless of the stage, as well as for the detection of small size metastases. Low price of the procedure, large accessibility and lack of the radiation, are among the most prominent advantages of CEUS that should be taken into consideration. Real time information and clinical character are among them also. These characteristics make CEUS a good and reliable procedure for the detection of liver tumors and follow–up under treatment. However, CEUS is restricted and with low performance in every case where 2D is limited e.g. attenuation, intense liver steatosis, deep region of interest. The procedure is limited to a single lesion and should be repeated to each other one when multiple tumors are detected. Finally, CEUS is operator and equipment dependent. These are reasons because CEUS cannot replace CT or MRI. In every case when the investigation is considered inconclusive, which happens in about 10 % of the cases, other sectional explorations must be considered, like the CT or MRI, and/or liver biopsy [48].

Abbreviations

US = ultrasonography; CEUS = contrast-enhanced ultrasonography; CA = contrast agent; HCC = hepatocellular carcinoma; CCC = cholangiocarcinoma; AP = accustic power;

Acknowledgements

The data presented into this chapter belong to the Research Program CEEX 138/2006 - Angiotumor financed by the Minister of Education & Research in România.

Author details

R. Badea[1] and Simona Ioaniţescu[2]

1 Department of Ultrasonography, 3rd Medical Clinic, "Octavian Fodor" Regional Institute of Gastroenterology and Hepatology, "Iuliu Hatieganu" University of Medicine and Pharmacy, Cluj-Napoca, Romania

2 Internal Medicine Centre, Fundeni Clinical Institute, Bucharest, Romania

References

[1] Hertzberg BS, Kliewer MA, Bowie JD et al. Physician training requirements in sonography: how many cases are needed for competence? AJR 2000; 174: 1 221 – 1 227

[2] Molins GI, Font FMJ, Alvaro JCA, Navarro JLL, Gil MF, Rodriguez CMF. Contrast – enhanced ultrasound in diagnosis and characterizarion of focal hepatic lesions. World J Radiol 2010, 28; 2 (12): 455 – 462

[3] Hoppmann R, Cook T, Hunt P, Fowler S, Paulman L, Wells J, Richeson N, Thomas L, Wilson B, Neuffer F, McCallum J, Smith S. Ultrasound in medical education: a vertical curriculum at the University of South Carolina School of Medicine. J S C Med Assoc. 2006 Dec;102(10):330-4

[4] Badea R, Badea Gh. Sonographische Untersuchungen des Pfortadersystems bei Lebertumoren. Ultraschall 1991; 12 (6): 272 – 276

[5] Rubin RA, Mitchell DG. Evaluation of the solid hepatic mass. Med Clin North Am 1996; 80: 907-928

[6] Bruneton JN, Raffaelli C, Balu-Maestro C, Padovani B, Chevallier P, Mourou MY. Sonographic diagnosis of solitary solid liver nodules in cancer patients. Eur Radiol 1996; 6: 439-442

[7] Ohlsson B, Nilsson J, Stenram U, Akerman M, Tranberg KG. Percutaneous fine-needle aspiration cytology in the diagnosis and management of liver tumours. Br J Surg 2002; 89: 757-762

[8] Bolondi L, Gaiani S, Celli N, Golfieri R, Grigioni WF, Leoni S, et al. Characterization of small nodules in cirrhosis by assessment of vascularity: the problem of hypovascular hepatocellular carcinoma. Hepatology 2005;42:27–34.

[9] Ando E, Kuromatsu R, Tanaka M, Takada A, Fukushima N, Sumie S, Nagaoka S, Akiyoshi J, Inoue K, Torimura T. Surveillance program for early detection of hepatocellular carcinoma in Japan: results of specialized department of liver disease. J Clin Gastroenterol. 2006;40:942-948

[10] Friedrich-Rust M, Ong MF, Herrmann E, Dries V, Samaras P, Zeuzem S, Sarrazin C. Real-Time Elastography for Noninvasive Assessment of Liver Fibrosis in Chronic Viral Hepatitis. AJR 2007; 188:758–764

[11] Lupsor M, Badea R, Stefănescu H, Grigorescu M, Sparchez Z, Serban A, Branda H, Iancu S, Maniu A. Analysis of Histopathological Changes that Influence Liver Stiffness in Chronic Hepatitis C. Results from a Cohort of 324 Patients. J Gastrointestin Liver Dis 2008; 17 (2): 155-163

[12] Lupsor M, Badea R, Stefanescu H, Sparchez Z, Branda H, Serban A, Maniu A. Performance of a new elastographic method (ARFI tehnology) compared to unidimensional transient elastography in the noninvasive assessment of chronic hepatitis C. Preliminary results. J Gastrointestin Liver Dis. 2009; 18 (3): 303-310

[13] Taylor KJW, Holland S. Doppler US. Part I. Basic principles, Instrumentation, and Pitfalls. Radiology 1990; 174:297 – 307

[14] McNaughton D.A, Abu-Yousef M.M. Doppler US of the Liver Made Simple. RadioGraphics 2011; 31:161–188. Published online 10.1148/rg.311105093 doi: 10.1148/rg.311105093

[15] Frinking PJ, Bouakaz A, Kirkhorn J, Ten Cate FJ, de Jong N. "Ultrasound contrast imaging: Current and new potential methods". Ultrasound Med Biol 2000; 26:965–975.

[16] Vicas C, Lupsor M, Badea R, Nedevschi S. Usefulness of textural analysis as a tool for noninvasive liver fibrosis staging. J Med Ultrasonics (2011) 38:105–117 DOI 10.1007/s10396-011-0307-x

[17] von Herbay A, Vogt C, Willers R, Häussinger D. Real-time imaging with the sonographic contrast agent SonoVue: differentiation between benign and malignant hepatic lesions. J Ultrasound Med 2004; 23: 1557-1568

[18] Quaia E. Microbubble ultrasound contrast agents: an update. Eur Radiol. 2007; 17: 1995–2008 DOI 10.1007/s00330-007-0623-0

[19] Forsberg F, Goldberg BB, Liu JB et al. Tissue specific US contrast agent for evaluation of hepatic and splenic parenchyma. Radiology 1999; 210:125–132

[20] D'Onofrio M, Martone E, Faccioli N, Zamboni G, Malago R, Pozzi Mucelli R. Focal liver lesions: sinusoidal phase of CEUS. Abdom Imaging. 2006; 31:529–536

[21] Wang YJ, Ng CK. The impact of quantitative imaging in medicine and surgery: Charting our course for the future. Quant Imaging Med Surg 2011;1:1-3. DOI: 10.3978/j.issn.2223-4292.2011.09.01

[22] Wilson SR, Burns PN. Microbubble-enhanced US in body imaging: what role? Radiology 2010; 257:24-39.

[23] Karhunen PJ. Benign hepatic tumours and tumour like conditions in men. J Clin Pathol 1986; 39:183–8

[24] Gibbs JF, Litwin AM, Kahlenberg MS. Contemporary management of benign liver tumors. Surg Clin N Am 84 (2004) 463 480

[25] Rubin RA, Mitchell DG. Evaluation of solid hepatic mass. Med Clin North Am 1996; 80:907 – 928

[26] Nicolau C, Vilana R, Catala V, Bianchi L, Gilabert R, Garcia A, Bru C. Importance of evaluating all vascular phases on contrast-enhanced sonography in the differentiation of benign from malignant focal liver lesions. Am J Roentgenol 2006; 186:158–167

[27] Wilson SR, Burns PN, Muradali D, Wilson JA, Lai X. Harmonic hepatic US with microbubble contrast agent: initial experience showing improved characterization of hemangioma, hepatocellular carcinoma, and metastasis. Radiology 2000; 215:153–161

[28] Pons F, Llovet JM. Approaching focal liver lesions. Rev Esp Enferm Dig 2004; 96: 567-573; 573-577

[29] Bartolotta TV, Taibbi A, Matranga D, Malizia G, Lagalla R, Midiri M. Hepatic focal nodular hyperplasia: contrast- enhanced ultrasound findings with emphasis on lesion size, depth and liver echogenicity. Eur Radiol. 2010; 20: 2248–2256

[30] Assy N, Nasser G, Djibre A, Beniashvili Z, Elias S, Zidan J. Characteristics of common solid liver lesions and recommendations for diagnostic workup. World J Gastroenterol 2009; 15: 3217-3227

[31] Parkin DM, Bray F, Ferlay J, Pisani P. Estimating the world cancer burden: Globocan 2000. Int J Cancer 2001; 94: 153-156

[32] Caturelli E, CastellanoL, Fusilli S, Palmentieri B, Niro GA, del Vecchio-Blanco C. Andriulli A, de Sio I. Coarse Nodular US Pattern in Hepatic Cirrhosis: Risk for Hepatocellular Carcinoma. Radiology 2003; 226:691–697

[33] International Working Party. Terminology of nodular hepatocellular lesions. Hepatology. 1995 Sep; 22 (3): 983 - 93.

[34] Kojiro M. "Nodule-in-nodule" appearance in hepatocellular carcinoma: its significance as a morphologic marker of dedifferentiation. Intervirology 2004; 47: 179-183.

[35] Kojiro M. Diagnostic discrepancy of early hepatocellular carcinoma between Japan and West. Hepatol Res 2007; 37 Suppl 2: S121-S124

[36] Kojiro M, Roskams T. Early hepatocellular carcinoma and dysplastic nodules. Semin Liver Dis 2005; 25: 133-142

[37] Ogata R, Majima Y, Tateishi Y, Kuromatsu R, Shimauchi Y, Torimyra T, Tanaka M, Kumashiro R, Kojiro M, Sata M. Bright loop appearance; a characteristic ultrasonography sign of early hepatocellular carcinoma. Oncol Rep 2000; 7: 1293-1298

[38] Tochio H, Kudo M. Afferent and efferent vessels of premalignant and overt hepatocellular carcinoma: observation by color Doppler imaging. Intervirology 2004; 47: 144-153

[39] Tochio H, Tomita S, Kudo M, Iwasaki N, Tamura S, Nakamura H, Soga T, Fukunaga T, Okabe Y, Kashida H, Hirasa M, Ibuki Y, Morimoto Y, Orino A. The efferent blood flow of early hepatocellular carcinoma and borderline lesions: Demonstration by color Doppler imaging. J Med Ultrason 2002; 29: 205-209

[40] Tarantino L, Francica G, Sordelli I et al. Diagnosis of benign and malig- nant portal vein thrombosis in cirrhotic patients with hepatocellular carcinoma: color Doppler US, contrast-enhanced US, and fine-needle biopsy. Abdom Imaging. 2006 Sep-Oct;31 (5): 537-44

[41] Nakajima T, Kondo Y, Miyazaki M, Okui K. A histopathologic study of 102 cases of intrahepatic cholangiocarcinoma: histologic classification and modes of spreading. Hum Pathol 1988; 19: 1228-1234

[42] Lim JH. Cholangiocarcinoma: morphologic classification according to growth pattern and imaging findings. Am J Roentgenol 2003; 181: 819-827

[43] Chen LD, Xu HX, Xie XY, Xie XH, Xu ZF, Liu GJ, Wang Z, Lin MX, Lu MD. Intrahepatic cholangiocarcinoma and he- patocellular carcinoma: differential diagnosis with contrast- enhanced ultrasound. Eur Radiol 2010; 20: 743-753

[44] Lazaridis G, Pentheroudakis G, Fountzilas G, Pavlidis N. Liver metastases from cancer of unknown primary (CUPL): a retrospective analysis of presentation, management and prog- nosis in 49 patients and systematic review of the literature. Cancer Treat Rev 2008; 34: 693-700

[45] Albrecht T, Blomley MJK, Burns PN et al. Improved detection of hepatic metastases with pulse-inversion US during the liver-specific phase of SHU 508A: multicenter study. Radiology 2003; 227:361–370

[46] Feier D, Socaciu M, Anton O, Al Hajjar N, Badea R. The combined role of intravenous contrast enhanced ultrasound (CEUS) and computed tomography (CT) in liver abscess diagnosis. Chirurgia (Bucur). 2012 May-Jun;107(3):343-51.

[47] Whittingham T. Contrast-specific imaging techniques: technical perspective. In: Quaia E (ed) Contrast media in ultrasonography: Basic principles and clinical applications. Springer, Berlin Heidelberg New York, 2005; pp 43–70

[48] Quaia E, Calliada F, Bertolotto M et al (2004) Characterization of focal liver lesions by contrast-specific US modes and a sulfur hexafluoride-filled microbubble contrast agent: diagnostic performance and confidence. Radiology 232:420–430

[49] Nicolau C, Vilana R, Catala V, Bianchi L, Gilabert R, Garcia A, Bru C. Importance of evaluating all vascular phases on contrast-enhanced sonography in the differentiation of benign from malignant focal liver lesions. Am J Roentgenol 2006; 186:158–167

Chapter 3

Role of Anti-Viral Therapy on Hepatitis B Virus (HBV)-Related Hepatocellular Carcinoma (HCC)

Charing Ching Ning Chong, Grace Lai Hung Wong,
Vincent Wai Sun Wong, Kit Fai Lee,
Paul Bo San Lai and Henry Lik Yuen Chan

Additional information is available at the end of the chapter

http://dx.doi.org/10.5772/55551

1. Introduction

Chronic hepatitis B virus (HBV) infection is a major global healthcare problem affecting around 350 million people. It can cause various complications including liver failure, hepatic decompensation and hepatocellular carcinoma (HCC), which lead to significant morbidity and mortality with more than 1 million deaths annually [1].

2. Epidemiology

HCC is one of the most common solid tumors worldwide. It is the fifth commonest cancer with more than 600 000 new cases per year. [2,3] It has been estimated that about 18,000 deaths occurred in the United States in 2008 because of cancer of the liver and intrahepatic bile ducts (mostly HCC), with a strong male preponderance as in Asian studies. [4] Although a certain proportion of these cases have been attributed to hepatitis C viral infection, it may be, at least in part, due to an increase in HBV-related HCC, particularly among immigrants from countries with high rates of endemic infection.

Many cohort studies in Asia have confirmed the high risk of HCC in HBsAg-positive individuals. [5,6] In a Chinese cohort with about 11,000 HBsAg-positive subjects followed over a mean period of 8 years, the relative risk of HCC in HBsAg-positive persons compared to HBsAg-negative controls was 18.8 for men and 33.2 for women. [6]

On the other hand, a long-term follow-up Italian study of apparently healthy blood donors found that only 0.6% of HBsAg-positive individuals developed HCC over an average period of follow-up of 29 years, which was no different from the 0.6% rate of HCC in a group of HBsAg-negative blood donor controls followed for a similar period of time. [7]

The reason(s) for this difference in HCC risk in HBsAg-positive individuals is not known. In general, HCC risk in HBsAg-positive individuals is determined partly by type of virus and timing of infection. In Asia, HBV infection is largely acquired by mother–child transmission while Western individuals usually acquire hepatitis B at an older age (adolescence or adulthood through sexual contact). Hence Western cohorts likely have shorter exposure and more successful immune clearance of hepatitis B than the typical Asian cohorts. Apart from the well-known environmental factors, individual genetic susceptibility also contributes to the risk of HCC. Some rare monogenic syndromes (e.g. alpha1-antitrypsin deficiency, hemochromatosis), as well as diseases inherited as polygenic traits (e.g. autoimmune hepatitis, a family history of HCC) are associated with a high risk of HCC. The genetic susceptibility to HCC is characterized by a genetic heterogeneity and caused by several unlinked single gene defects. [8]

3. Pathogenesis of HCC development in chronic HBV infection

Chronic HBV infection is the dominant cause of HCC in Asia because of the endemic status of HBV. Hepatic inflammation and cirrhosis also favor the process of carcinogenesis. The risk for HCC development is increased in patients with older age and liver cirrhosis [9]. Some viral characteristics, namely positive hepatitis B e antigen (HBeAg), high serum HBV DNA level, HBV genotypes and subgenotypes, and basal core promoter mutants, are associated with an increase risk of developing HCC. [9 – 12] The level of serum hepatitis B surface antigen (HBsAg), which is not affected by the antiviral drugs, is potentially a biomarker of viral persistence during antiviral therapy which may be a useful marker of HCC development. [13] The role of this and other biomarkers is discussed below.

3.1. Serum HBV DNA level

The risk of HCC is increased in patients with higher levels of HBV replication, one manifestation of which is high level of serum HBV DNA level. Several large prospective Asian studies found that high level of HBV DNA was an independent risk factor for the development of HCC. [11, 14] [Figure 1]

A famous Taiwanese REVEAL-HBV study (abbreviated from the Risk Evaluation of Viral Load Elevation and Associated Liver Disease/Cancer–Hepatitis B Virus) reported that the incidence of HCC increased with the serum HBV DNA strata. Among a cohort of 3,653 patients from the community, the cumulative incidence increased from 0.74% for patients with undetectable HBV DNA (<300 copies/ml) to 13.5% for those with HBV DNA ≥ 1,000, 000 more copies/ml at a mean follow-up of 11.4 years. [14]

In another prospective cohort study involving 1,006 Chinese patients in Hong Kong, the hazard ratios for HCC were 1.62 and 2.73 in those with serum HBV DNA 4.5-6.5 log copies/ml and above 6.5 log copies/ml respectively, compared to those of low viremia (<4.5 log copies/ml). [11]

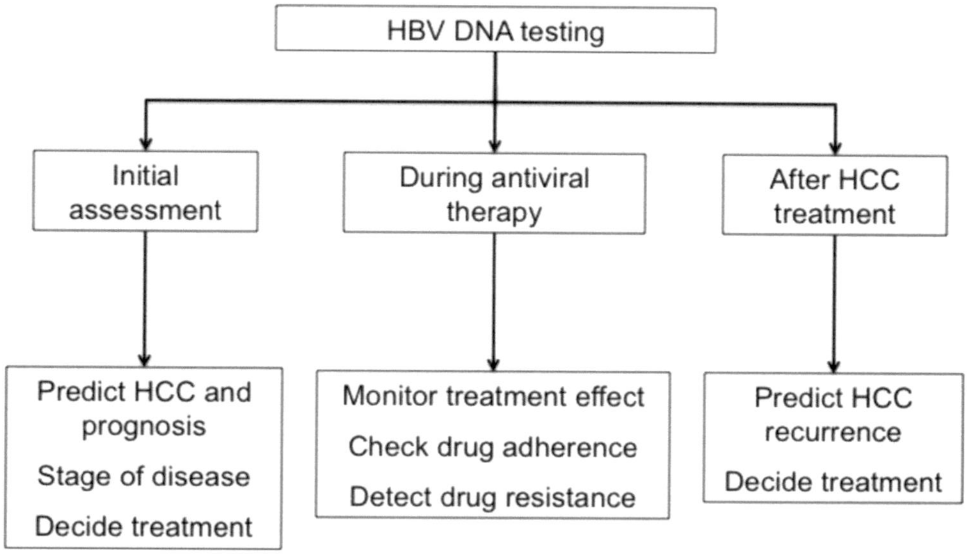

Figure 1. Role of HBV DNA testing

3.2. Hepatitis B e Antigen (HBeAg)

Hepatitis B e antigen (HBeAg) positivity is another manifestation of high levels of HBV replication. Compared to HBV non-carrier, the relative risk of HCC was increased as high as 60-fold among those positive for both HBsAg and HBeAg in a large prospective cohort study of 11 893 Taiwanese men. The relative risk was 6 times higher among HBeAg-positive patients than those who were HBeAg-negative. [10] Furthermore, clearance of HBeAg, whether spontaneous or after antiviral therapy, reduced the risk of hepatic decompensation, HCC occurrence and improved survival. [15, 16]

On the other hand, 10% to 30% of patients may still have elevated ALT and high HBV DNA levels after HBeAg seroconversion; 10% to 20% of inactive carriers may have reactivation of HBV replication and exacerbations of hepatitis after years of quiescence. [17, 18] These patients may still be at risk of HCC development.

3.3. Serum Quantitative Hepatitis B Surface Antigen (qHBsAg)

HBsAg level or qHBsAg reflects the transcriptional activity of covalently closed circular (ccc) DNA, the template for viral replication inside the nuclei of hepatocytes. [19] The combination of low serum qHBsAg and HBV DNA levels may be an accurate identification of "true inactive carriers" and prediction of HBsAg loss in the HBeAg-negative patients. [20] HBsAg level below

100 IU/ml can predict HBsAg loss over time in genotype B or C HBV-infected patients. [13] A recent Taiwanese study demonstrated that a high HBsAg level (≥ 1000 IU/mL) predicted the risk of HCC among patients with low serum HBV DNA level (< 2000 IU/mL). [21] In another prospective population-based cohort study with 1271 Alaskan natives with chronic HBV infection followed up for an average of 19.6 years, the incidence of HCC after clearance of HBsAg was significantly lower than the rate in those who remained HBsAg-positive. [22] However, despite the loss of HBsAg, HBV DNA was still detected in the sera of around 18% patient subjects after clearance. Hence, patients with chronic hepatitis B who have lost HBsAg can still develop HCC, even in the absence of cirrhosis. These patients should still be monitored regularly.

3.4. HBV genotypes and subgenotypes

Hepatitis B virus has been classified into at least 10 genotypes on the basis of an intergroup divergence of 8% or more in the complete genome nucleotide sequence. [23, 24] HBV subgenotypes are also identified within some genotypes such as subgenotype Ce and Cs in genotype C [11]. Compared to HBV genotype B, genotype C is associated with a 2- to 3-fold increase in risk of HCC development; [25] whereas HBV subgenotype Ce has the highest risk of HCC (hazard ratio = 2.75) and HBV subgenotype Cs has intermediate risk (hazard ratio = 1.70). [11]

One of the reasons of the increased risks in genotype C is that more patients infected with this genotype have persistently positive HBeAg and fluctuating HBeAg whereas more patients infected with genotype B HBV have persistently negative HBeAg. [25] This reflects a relatively higher level of viremia among patients infected with genotype C [26]. Due to prolonged immune clearance phase, more patients with genotype C infection eventually develop cirrhosis. [19]

The effect of genotype C and high HBV DNA level may be an independent direct pathway of hepatocarcinogenesis on top of liver cirrhosis, which is the result of continuous necroinflammation. [27] Increased cis-activation of the proto-oncogene, suppression of tumor suppressor gene, or transactivation by the HBV X protein are additional carcinogenic mechanisms. [28, 29]

3.5. Basal core promoter mutations

Basal core promoter mutations (A to T at nucleotide 1762 and G to A at nucleotide 1764), which are commonly found in HBV genotype C, may increase the risk of HCC development. [30] However, the prevalence of basal core promoter mutations increases with HBeAg seroconversion. [31, 32] In a longitudinal study of 426 patients, there was no independent association between basal core mutations and HCC development after adjustment for genotype C and serum HBV DNA level. [25]

4. Risk factors of HBV-related HCC recurrence

Although liver resection is the treatment of choice for early HCC, the 5-year overall survival after tumor resection is in the region of only 55%. [33, 34] The annual recurrence rate of HCC is 15% to 20%, with a cumulative 5-year recurrence rate of up to 70% after curative resection. [35] High levels of recurrence after tumor resection are associated with mortality. [36]

There are two distinct types of HCC recurrence: early and late recurrence. Early recurrence describes that arising from dissemination of the primary tumor, which usually occurs within the first one to two years after the curative treatment. Early recurrence is often associated with some tumor characteristics such as multi-nodularity of the tumour and a smaller surgical margin of normal liver at the time of resection. [37]

Late recurrence is often related to the development of *de novo* HCC arising from a "field effect" in the diseased liver, which may be related to viral effects as well as the severity of liver fibrosis. [38] Hence the risk factors of late recurrence may be similar to those of HCC development, namely presence of liver cirrhosis, high serum HBV DNA level and genotype C and high alanine aminotransferase (ALT). [39-42] (Table 1)

Risk Factors for HCC Recurrence	
EARLY RECURRENCE	LATE RECURRENCE
History of Rupture	High serum HBV DNA level
Presence of lymphovascular permeation	High serum alanine aminotransferase (ALT) level
Macro- or micro-vascular invasion	Genotype C
Multifocal lesions	Liver cirrhosis
High AFP level	High Ishak hepatic inflammatory activity
Close surgical margin	High ICG-15
	Multifocal lesions

Table 1. Risk Factors for HCC Recurrence

5. Role of antiviral therapy in HBV-related HCC

Patients with HBV-related HCC suffer not only from malignancy but also chronic HBV infection. These two conditions interact with each other such that treatments for HCC may affect the activity of viral replication, whereas treatments for chronic HBV infection may influence the clinical outcome of HCC.

The association between high serum HBV load and increased risk of HCC and liver cirrhosis had been demonstrated by many studies. [14, 43] The high serum HBV DNA load is not only a key risk factor for the development and recurrence of HCC, but also the risk factor that is most amenable to control.

Antiviral therapy for HBV includes nucleos(t)ide analogs (e.g. lamivudine, adefovir, entecavir, tenofovir and telbivudine) and (peg)interferon. [44] They are all shown to achieve persistent viral suppression short term, which theoretically can retard HBV reactivation, reduce HCC occurrence and ultimately prolong patient survival.

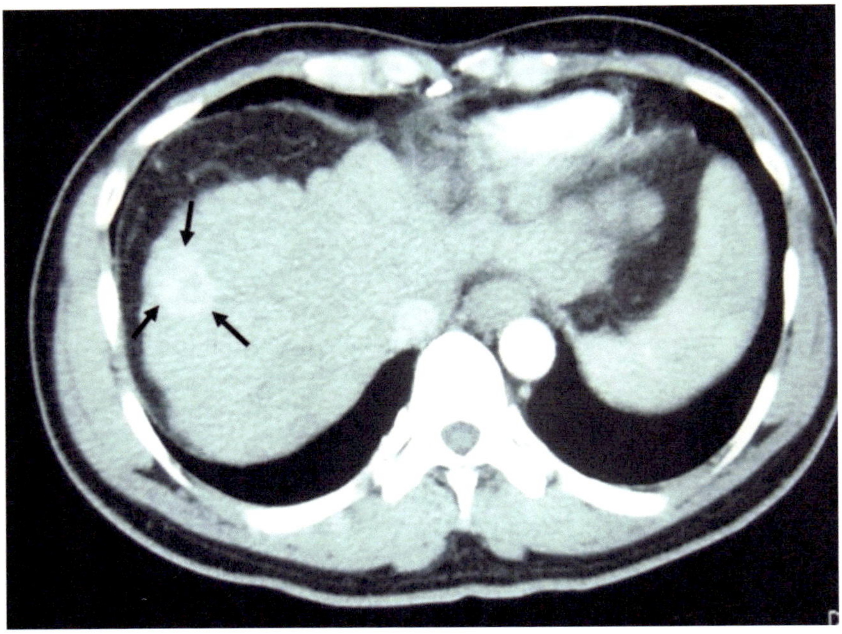

Figure 2. Computer tomography image showing a very cirrhotic liver with HCC

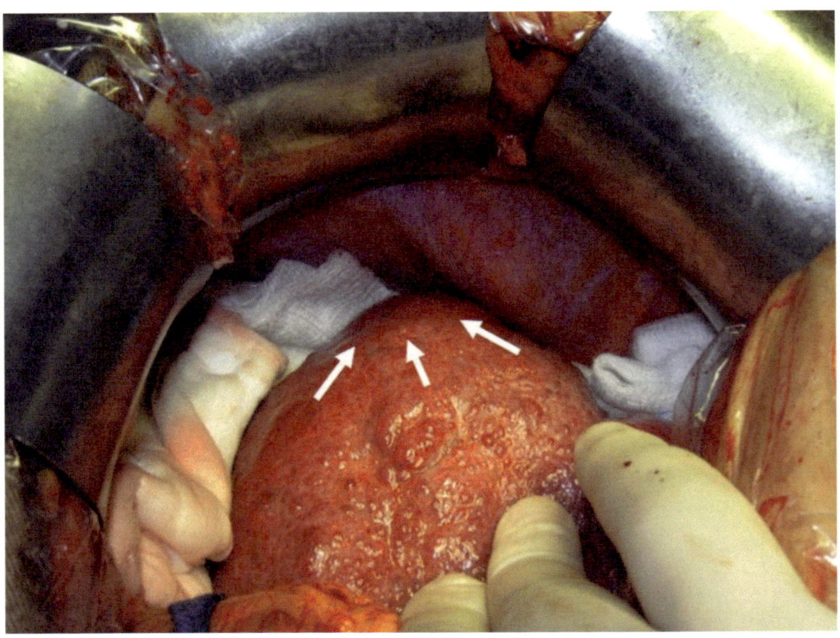

Figure 3. Intra-operative picture of a patient with HCC developed in a background of macronodular liver cirrhosis

5.1. Antiviral therapy to prevent HBV-related HCC development

High serum HBV DNA levels have been shown to be associated with an increased risk of cirrhosis and HCC. [Figure 2, 3] Moreover, in a large prospective study of more than 3000 patients with a mean follow-up of 11.4 years, Chen et al found that the incidence of HCC correlated with serum HBV DNA level at time of enrollment. Furthermore, in the sub-analysis, spontaneous decline of viremia levels was associated with a reduced risk of HCC development by comparison with patients who maintained high viremia levels. [13] In their conclusion, the authors emphasized the effective control of HBV replication with antiviral therapy in order to reduce the risk of HCC.

As persistent viral replication is associated with development of HCC, antiviral therapy effective in viral suppression may reduce HCC occurrence. Results from randomized controlled trials and multicenter retrospective studies have shown that continuous treatment with nucleos(t)ide analogues in patients with chronic hepatitis B or cirrhosis reduce the risk of HCC development. [16, 45]

Nucleoside analog lamivudine reduced the risk of HCC development by 50% compared to placebo in a randomized controlled trial involving 651 patients. [16] Unfortunately the beneficial effect of nucleos(t)ide analog may be decreased with the emergence of drug resistance mutations, namely tyrosine, methionine, aspartate (YMDD) mutations. [46] New generation nucleos(t)ide analogs of lower risk of drug resistance mutation would potentially benefit HBV-infected patients more.

Interferon-alpha (IFN-α) was the first agent approved by the Food and Drug Administration for chronic HBV infection in the 1980s. [47] Peginterferon-alpha (pIFN-α) was produced by the addition of a polyethylene glycol moiety to interferon. Consequently pIFN-α has longer half-life and higher average concentration in the body, and is now widely used due to the convenient weekly dosing. [48] Unlike oral antiviral agents, (p)IFN-α is given for finite treatment duration and administrated subcutaneously. A few meta-analyses have suggested a reduced risk of HCC and other liver-related events after (p)IFN-α treatment. [46, 48] The risk of HCC after (p)IFN-α treatment has been reportedly reduced by 34%, with the benefit is more significant among patients with early cirrhosis than among those without cirrhosis. [46]

5.2. Antiviral therapy to prevent HBV reactivation of HCC patients

Treatments for HCC, including surgical resection, local ablative therapies, transarterial chemoembolization (TACE), may affect the activity of HBV replication, a factor that has important implications for hepatitis activity. If the treatments subsequently lead to HBV reactivation, the patient outcome may be jeopardized. [49] Most of the data on this aspect came from several studies concerning HCC patients received TACE, which involves the administration of chemotherapeutic agents targeted to the liver and raises the concern about HBV reactivation. There is a degree of inconsistency, however, with some previous studies contradicting this risk of HBV reactivation after TACE. [50, 51] A more recent study demonstrated that high-level treatment intensity, together with high HBV DNA level, was the major risk factor for HBV reactivation during TACE. [52]

HBV may also reactivate in the peri-operative period after liver resection for HCC, even among patients with relatively low HBV DNA level (<200 IU/ml). [53] This phenomenon may be explained by the fact that a single HBV DNA level at a given time is not always indicative of permanent immune-suppression of HBV replication, as indicated particularly by more recent analyses of the REVEAL data. [54]

Studies reported that an effective pre-operative anti-HBV therapy could contribute to an improvement in liver function. In a recent Chinese study, Huang et al found that hepatitis B e antigen (HBeAg) positivity, preoperative HBV-DNA above the lower limit of quantification (≥200 IU/mL), Ishak inflammation score of greater than 3, preoperative TACE, operation time of more than 180 minutes, blood transfusion, and without prophylactic antiviral therapy were significantly associated with an increased risk of HBV reactivation. More importantly, this study showed that the 3-year disease-free survival (DFS) rate and overall survival (OS) rates after resection in patients with HBV reactivation were significantly lower than those without reactivation. Another study by Thia et al reported the incidence of all causes of post-operative hepatitis and the exacerbation of chronic hepatitis B. [55] In this study, 1- and 2-year survival rates were poorest for the ECHB group at 42.9 and 21.4%, compared with those with postoperative hepatitis due to other causes at 60.3 and 45.2% and those without postoperative hepatitis at 87.7 and 73.5%, and the difference were statistically significant. As a result, the authors recommended routine prophylactic antiviral treatment before partial hepatectomy.

The use of nucleos(t)ide analogs such as lamivudine may be useful to reduce the risk of HBV reactivation related to TACE or liver resection. [53, 56]

5.3. Antiviral therapy to prevent HBV-related HCC recurrence after curative treatment

As discussed above, tumour recurrence after curative treatment of HCC was increased with the level of HBV DNA and alanine aminotransferase (ALT). [41, 42] This implies that HBV viral replication may play an important role in HCC development and high rates of viral replication are positively associated with a high risk of HCC recurrence after surgery. As antiviral therapy is effective in reducing HCC development, it is logical to believe that it can also reduce HCC recurrence after curative treatment.

Results from currently available reports were not conclusive. In a small Hong Kong study, Hung et al studied 72 patients who underwent hepatectomy for HCC and found that patients with high viral load (greater than 2000IU/mL) had a significantly higher risk of HCC recurrence after resection and viral load was the most important correctable risk factor for post-hepatectomy HCC recurrence. [40] However, the impressive result should be interpreted with caution, as the number of patients treated with antiviral therapy in this study was small.

A Korean group also reported similar findings in a cohort study of 157 patients. [57] The 5-year cumulative recurrence rates of 68 viremic patients were compared with that of another 89 non-viremic patients. The 5-year cumulative recurrence rate was significantly higher in the viremic group (73%) compared with 55% in the non-viremic group and persistent viremia was an independent risk factor for increased recurrence after surgery. The authors concluded that antiviral therapy should be initiated in those with detectable serum HBV DNA in order to prevent long-term recurrences.

However, these results could not be reproduced in other studies. A recent comparative study by the Chinese group involving 79 patients with a median follow-up of 12 months showed no significant difference in the recurrence rate after surgery in the treatment and control group. [58] The cumulative recurrence rates of HCC did not differ significantly between a group treated with lamivudine and the control group in a Japanese study. [59] However, Kuzuya did report that all patients in the lamivudine group were able to receive curative treatment for recurrent HCC while 10 of 15 patients in the control group were unable to receive curative optimal therapy for recurrent HCC due to deterioration in remnant liver function.

Two meta-analyses have explored this issue. Miao reported that postoperative antiviral therapy as a whole has been shown to reduce HCC recurrence at year 1, 2, 3, and 5. [60] Another meta-analysis by Wong et al demonstrated that nucleos(t)ide analogue treatment was beneficial in reducing the risk of HCC recurrence after curative treatment for 41%. [61] [Table 2]

Study	Treated with antiviral		Untreated		OR, 95% C.I.
	Total	Events	Total	Events	
Li 2010	43	33	36	33	0.30 [0.08, 1.19]
Koda 2009	22	17	14	12	0.57 [0.09, 3.42]
Chuma 2009	20	8	64	22	1.27 [0.45, 3,57]
Hung 2008	10	0	62	30	0.05 [0.00, 0.90]
Yoshida 2008	33	18	71	40	0.93 [0.41, 2.13]
Kuzuya 2007	16	7	33	15	0.93 [0.28, 3.11]
Kubo 2007	14	2	10	5	0.17 [0.02, 1.16]
Shuqun 2006	16	14	17	17	0.17 [0.01, 3.73]
Piao 2005	30	14	40	26	0.47 [0.18, 1.19]

Table 2. The summary of studies comparing the effect of anti-viral treatment vs no treatment in hepatocellular carcinoma recurrence

The effect of (p)IFN-α treatment in prevention of HBV-related HCC recurrence was found controversial in a meta-analysis and systemic review. [62, 63] In addition, use of (p)IFN-α in HCC patients may be risky as they are more vulnerable to the development of hepatic decompensation with life-threatening complications including hepatic encephalopathy, ascites *etc.* [64]

In contrast, nucleos(t)ide analogues are safe and better tolerated than (p)IFN-α. Results from a randomized controlled trial [16] and multicentre retrospective study [45] have shown that continuous treatment with a nucleotide analogue in patients with chronic hepatitis B or cirrhosis can reduce the risk of HCC development.

5.4. Antiviral therapy to improve survival after curative treatment of HBV-related HCC

Antiviral treatment may render patients with HBV-related HCC able to tolerate HCC treatments better and may improve prognosis. However, the currently available studies on whether antiviral therapy is beneficial to the survival after treatment for HCC are limited.

In the Kuzuya et al study, although there was no significant difference in the survival rate between the two groups, the survival rates in the lamivudine group tended to be higher than those in the control group ($p = 0.063$). [59]

Similar findings were reported in a RCT by Liaw et al. [16] Although they did not show a significant effect of lamivudine on HCC recurrence, there was a significant benefit in the overall survival. They suggested that continuous treatment with lamivudine would lead to a delay in clinical progression in patients with chronic hepatitis B and advanced fibrosis or cirrhosis by a significant reduction in the incidence of hepatic decompensation and risk of HCC.

Li et al, in a recent nonrandomized study, compared the impact of antiviral treatment in 79 patients who underwent curative hepatectomy for HCC. [58] Forty-three patients received lamivudine with or without adefovir as treatment and had a significantly higher HBeAg seroconversion rate compared with the 36 patents in the control group who received no antiviral treatment. This study showed the efficacy of post-operative antiviral therapy in suppressing viral replication and hence the authors suggested the initiation of antiviral treatment in patients with detectable serum HBV DNA level after resection. Furthermore, Li et al reported a significantly greater improvement in the residual liver volume per unit surface area at 6 months after hepatectomy in the anti-viral therapy group. [58] Remnant liver function is a major determining factor in selecting subsequent treatment for HCC recurrence and is a key prognostic factor for the overall survival. Therefore, a higher chance of receiving aggressive salvage therapy during HCC recurrence could be observed among patients receiving antiviral therapy due to better liver reserve, and resulting in a better survival. [40, 59]

The previously mentioned meta-analysis reported that antiviral therapy significantly improved overall survival, as both the mortality related to liver failure and the overall mortality were reduced. The improvement in survival was contributed to by the reduction of HCC recurrence as well as the improvement in liver function after antiviral therapy. [60] Previous studies have shown that lamivudine and telbivudine therapy could effectively suppress the HBV DNA level and improve the liver function in patients with decompensated cirrhosis. [65-67] [Table 3]

These results are particularly important because up to now, there has been no effective adjuvant treatment to prevent HCC recurrence. There is no proven role for adjuvant chemotherapy or transarterial chemo-embolization (TACE), [68] while the result for molecular targeted chemotherapy is awaited.

Although there is not enough data to suggest nucleos(t)ide analogs would reduce short-term recurrence rate or progression of disease, the enhanced post-operative viral clearance, improved residual liver volume, and promoted hepatocyte regeneration in HCC patients with

http://dx.doi.org/10.5772/55551

Study	Treated with antiviral		Untreated		OR, 95% C.I.
	Total	Events	Total	Events	
Li 2010	43	41	36	36	0.23 [0.01, 4.89]
Koda 2009	22	4	14	7	0.22 [0.05, 1.00]
Hung 2008	10	0	62	7	0.35 [0.02, 6.65]
Yoshida 2008	33	8	71	32	0.39 [0.15, 0.98]
Kuzuya 2007	16	0	33	6	0.13 [0.01, 2.43]
Kubo 2007	14	0	10	3	0.07 [0.00, 1.63]
Shuqun 2006	16	15	17	17	0.30 [0.01, 7.79]
Piao 2005	30	2	40	12	0.17 [0.03. 0.81]

Table 3. The summary of studies comparing the effect of anti-viral treatment vs. no treatment in the overall mortality of hepatocellular carcinoma

active hepatitis B, may significantly improve the tolerance to subsequent therapy. Hopefully, this would translate into an improvement in the overall survival.

Role of antiviral therapy as an adjuvant therapy after curative treatment of HCC should be a great topic for future studies. Further studies with more patients and longer follow-up are necessary to clarify the efficacy of antiviral treatment on HBV load and, more importantly, on survival for HBV-related HCC patients who undergo hepatectomy.

6. Drawbacks of antiviral therapy

The main drawback of the long-term use of anti-viral therapy is the emergence of drug resistance, especially for lamivudine, whose reported resistance is about 14% to 39%. [58-59, 69-70] Newer nucleotide analogues with lower resistance rates currently recommended by international guidelines may provide better viral suppression and potentially even better long-term outcomes. [71-73] Road- map models using lamivudine or telbivudine as first line agents were recently found to be a cost-effective approach for HBeAg-positive patients in Asia, while entecavir and tenofovir monotherapies were more cost-effective than the roadmap models in HBeAg-negative patients. [74] These guidelines may also be considered in HCC patients.

7. Future development

The main goal of antiviral therapy for chronic hepatitis B is to prevent the development of liver cirrhosis and HCC. Unfortunately, although many guidelines for the treatment of chronic hepatitis B have been commenced, global guideline for the use of antiviral treatment on HBV-related HCC is lacking so far. According to the American Association for the Study of Liver Diseases and Asian Pacific Association for the Study of the Liver guidelines, the factors for initiating antiviral treatments include high serum HBV DNA levels (greater than 105 copies/ml), high ALT levels (more than 2 x ULN) and presence of biopsy-confirmed liver disease or cirrhosis. [75, 76] [Table 4]

HBeAg	HBV DNA (PCR)	ALT	Recommended Treatment
Positive	≥20 000 IU/ml	≤ 2X ULN	Low efficacy with current treatment. Observe; consider treatment when ALT becomes elevated. Consider biopsy in persons ≥ 40 years, ALT persistently high normal – 2X ULN, or with family history of HCC. Consider treatment if HBV DNA ≥ 20 000 IU/ml and biopsy shows moderate/severe inflammation or significant fibrosis.
Positive	≥20 000 IU/ml	≥ 2X ULN	Observe for 3-6 months and treat if no spontaneous HBeAg loss. Consider liver biopsy prior to treatment if compensated. Immediate treatment if icteric or clinical decompensation. IFN-α / pIFN-α, LAM, ADV, ETV or LdT may be used as initial therapy. LAM and LdT not preferred due to high rate of drug resistance. End-point of treatment – Seroconversion from HBeAg to anti-HBe. Duration of therapy: IFN-α: 16 weeks pIFN-α: 48 weeks LAM/ADV/ETV/LdT: minimum 1 year, continue for at least 6 months after HBeAg sero-conversion. IFN-α non-responders / contraindications to IFN-α → ADV/ETV.
Negative	≥20 000 IU/ml	≥ 2X ULN	IFN-α / pIFN-α, LAM, ADV, ETV or LdT may be used as initial therapy, LAM and LdT not preferred due to high rate of drug resistance. End-point of treatment – not defined. Duration of therapy: IFN-α/pIFN-α: 1 year LAM/ADV/ETV/LdT: ≥ 1 year IFN-α non-responders / contraindications to IFN-α → ADV/ETV.
Negative	≥2 000 IU/ml	1 - ≥ 2X ULN	Consider liver biopsy and treat if liver biopsy shows moderate/severe necro-inflammation or significant fibrosis.
Negative	≤ 2 000 IU/ml	≤ ULN	Observe, treat if HBV DNA or ALT becomes higher.
Equivocal	Detectable	Cirrhosis	Compensated: HBV DNA ≥ 2 000 IU/ml – Treat, LAM/ADV/ETV/LdT may be used as initial therapy. LAM and LdT not preferred due to high rate of drug resistance. Decompensated: Coordinate treatment with transplant center, LAM (or LdT) + ADV or ETV preferred. Refer for liver transplant
Equivocal	Detectable	Cirrhosis	Compensated: Observe. Decompensated: Refer for liver transplant.

Abbreviations: ALT, alanine. aminotransferase; ULN, upper limit of normal; IFN-α, interferon alpha; pIFN-α, pegylated IFN-alpha; LAM, lamivudine; ADV, adefovir; ETV, entecavir; LdT, telbivudine

Table 4. American Association for the Study of Liver Diseases and Asian Pacific Association for the Study of Liver recommendations for treatment of chronic hepatitis B

Development of HCC is not included in the consideration of antiviral treatment. However, late recurrence is mostly due to de novo carcinogenesis associated with HBV viremia as well as the "field effect" in HBV-related HCC. The use of anti-HBV treatment as adjuvant therapy after the resection or ablation of HCC for the patients with a high HBV DNA level to prevent late recurrence should be revisited, given that the incidence of recurrence is higher than that of the initial HCC development. [77]

In the future, we look forward to more randomized studies with larger sample size, longer follow-up periods, with regular monitoring of HBV DNA. These data will help to clarify the beneficial effects of antiviral therapies in HCC, in particular if there should be a lower threshold for commencing antiviral treatment to prevent HBV-related HCC.

8. Conclusions

There is increasing evidence showing the potential beneficial effects of the antiviral therapy in reducing the HBV viral load, preventing reactivation of HBV and improving survival of HBV-related HCC patients. Anti-viral therapy with nucleotide analogues may be preferable than interferon treatment due to less adverse side effects and can be considered as a cost-effective adjuvant therapy for HCC after curative treatment. Confirmatory prospective studies with larger sample size and longer follow-up period are awaited.

Author details

Charing Ching Ning Chong[1], Grace Lai Hung Wong[2], Vincent Wai Sun Wong[2], Kit Fai Lee[1], Paul Bo San Lai[1] and Henry Lik Yuen Chan[2]

1 Division of Hepato-biliary and Pancreatic Surgery, Department of Surgery, Prince of Wales Hospital, the Chinese University of Hong Kong, Hong Kong, SAR, China

2 Institute of Digestive Disease and Department of Medicine & Therapeutics, Prince of Wales Hospital, the Chinese University of Hong Kong, Hong Kong, SAR, China

References

[1] Chan HLY, Sung JJY. Hepatocellular carcinoma and hepatitis B virus. Seminars in Liver Disease 2006;26(2) 153-161.

[2] McGlynn KA, London WT. Epidemiology and natural history of hepatocellular carcinoma. Best Practice and Reseach. Clinical Gastroenterology 2005;19(1) 3-23.

[3] Sherman M. Hepatocellular carcinoma: epidemiology, risk factors, and screening. Seminars in Liver Disease 2005;25(2) 43-154.

[4] Jemal A, Siegel R, Ward E, Hao Y, Xu J, Murray T, Thun MJ. Cancer Statistics, 2008. CA: a Cancer Journal for Clinicians 2008;58(2) 71-96.

[5] Beasley RP, Hwang LY, Lin CC, Chien C-S. Hepatocellular carcinoma and hepatitis B virus: a prospective study of 22,707 men in Taiwan. Lancet 1981;2(8256) 1129-1133.

[6] Evans A, Chen GH, Ross E, Shen FM, Lin WY, London W. Eight-year follow-up of the 90,000-person Haimen City cohort: I. Hepatocellular carcinoma mortality, risk factors, and gender differences. Cancer Epidemiology, Biomarkers and Prevention 2002;11(4) 369-376.

[7] Manno M, Camma C, Schepis F, Bassi F, Gelmini R, Giannini F, Miselli F, Grottola A, Ferretti I, Vecchi C, De Palma M, Villa E. Natural history of chronic HBV carriers in Northern Italy: morbidity and mortality after 30 years. Gastroenterology 2004;127(3) 756-763.

[8] Dragani TA. Risk of HCC: genetic heterogeneity and complex genetics. J Hepatol. 2010;52:252-7.

[9] Wong VWS, Chan SL, Mo F, Chan TC, Loong HH, Wong GL, Lui YY, Chan AT, Sung JJ, Yeo W, Chan HL, Mok TS. Clinical scoring system to predict hepatocellular carcinoma in chronic hepatitis B carriers. Journal of Clinical Oncology 2010;28(10) 1660-1665.

[10] Yang HI, Lu SN, Liaw YF, You SL, Sun CA, Wang LY, Hsiao CK, Chen PJ, Chen DS, Chen CJ; Taiwan Community-Based Cancer Screening Project Group. Hepatitis B e antigen and the risk of hepatocellular carcinoma. New England Journal of Medicine 2002; 347(3) 168-174.

[11] Chan HLY, Tse CH, Mo F, Koh J, Wong VW, Wong GL, Lam Chan S, Yeo W, Sung JJ, Mok TS. High viral load and hepatitis B virus subgenotype Ce are associated with increased risk of hepatocellular carcinoma. Journal of Clinical Oncology 2008; 26(2) 177-182.

[12] Chan HLY. JGH Foundation emerging leadership lecture. Significance of hepatitis B virus genotypes and mutations in the development of hepatocellular carcinoma in Asia. Journal of Gastroenterology and Hepatology 2011;26(1) 8-12.

[13] Chan HLY, Wong GLH, Tse CH, Chan HY, Wong VM. Viral determinants of hepatitis B surface antigen seroclearance in hepatitis B e antigen negative chronic hepatitis B patients. The Journal of Infectious Disease 2011;204(3) 408-414.

[14] Chen CJ, Yang HI, Su J, Jen CL, You SL, Lu SN, Huang GT, Iloeje UH; REVEAL-HBV Study Group. Risk of hepatocellular carcinoma across a biological gradient of serum hepatitis B virus DNA Level. Journal of the American Medical Association, 2006;295(1) 65–73.

[15] de Jongh FE, Janssen HL, de Man RA, Hop WC, Schalm SW, van Blankenstein M. Survival and prognostic indicators in hepatitis B surface antigen-positive cirrhosis of the liver. Gastroenterology 1992;103(5):1630-1635.

[16] Liaw YF, Sung JJ, Chow WC, Farrell G, Lee CZ, Yuen H, Tanwandee T, Tao QM, Shue K, Keene ON, Dixon JS, Gray DF, Sabbat J; Cirrhosis Asian Lamivudine Multicentre Study Group. Lamivudine for patients with chronic hepatitis B and advanced liver disease. N Engl J Med 2004;351:1521-31.

[17] Lok AS, Lai CL. Acute exacerbations in Chinese patients with chronic hepatitis B virus (HBV) infection. Incidence, predisposing factors and etiology. Journal of Hepatology 1990;10(1) 29-34.

[18] Hsu YS, Chien RN, Yeh CT, Sheen IS, Chiou HY, Chu CM, Liaw YF. Long-term outcome after spontaneous HBeAg seroconversion in patients with chronic hepatitis B. Hepatology 2002;35(6) 1522-1527.

[19] Chan HLY, Wong VWS, Tse AML, Tse CH, Chim AM, Chan HY, Wong GL, Sung JJ. Serum hepatitis B surface antigen quantitation can reflect hepatitis B virus in the liver and predict treatment response. Clinical Gastroenterology and Hepatology 2007;5(12) 1462–1468.

[20] Chan HLY, Thompson A, Martinot-Peignoux M, Piratvisuth T, Cornberg M, Brunetto MR, Tillmann HL, Kao JH, Jia JD, Wedemeyer H, Locarnini S, Janssen HL, Marcellin P. Hepatitis B surface antigen quantification: why and how to use it in 2011 - a core group report. Journal of Hepatology 2011;55(5) 1121-1131.

[21] Tseng TC, Liu CJ, Yang HC, Su TH, Wang CC, Chen CL, Kuo SF, Liu CH, Chen PJ, Chen DS, Kao JH. High levels of hepatitis B surface antigen increase risk of hepatocellular carcinoma in patients with low HBV load. Gastroenterology 2012;142(5) 1140-1149.e3.

[22] Simonetti J, Bulkow L, McMahon BJ, Homan C, Snowball M, Negus S, Williams J, Livingston SE. Clearance of hepatitis B surface antigen and risk of hepatocellular carcinoma in a cohort chronically infected with hepatitis B virus. Hepatology 2010;51(5) 1531-1537.

[23] Wong GLH, Chan HLY. Molecular virology in chronic hepatitis B: genotypes. Hospital Medicine 2005;66(1) 13-16.

[24] Lin CL, Kao JH. The clinical implications of hepatitis B virus genotype: recent advances. Journal of Gastroenterology and Hepatology 2011; 26(Suppl 1):123–130.

[25] Chan HLY, Hui AY, Wong ML, Tse AM, Hung LC, Wong VW, Sung JJ. Genotype C hepatitis B virus infection is associated with an increased risk of hepatocellular carcinoma. Gut 2004;53(10) 1494-1498.

[26] Chan HLY, Wong ML, Hui AY, Hung LC, Chan FK, Sung JJ. The value of hepatitis B virus DNA quantitation to predict hepatitis B e antigen reversion in chronic hepatitis B. Journal of Clinical Microbiology 2003; 41(10) 4693-4695.

[27] Ohkubo K, Kato Y, Ichikawa T, Kajiya Y, Takeda Y, Higashi S, Hamasaki K, Nakao K, Nakata K, Eguchi K. Viral load is a significant prognostic factor for hepatitis B virus-associated hepatocellular carcinoma. Cancer 2002;94(10) 2663-2668.

[28] Shafritz DA, Kew MC. Identification of integrated hepatitis B virus DNA sequences in human hepatocellular carcinoma. Hepatology. 1981;1(1) 1-8.

[29] Matsubara K, Tokino T. Integration of hepatitis B virus DNA and its implications for hepatocarcanogenesis. Molecular Biology and Medicine 1990;7(3) 243-260.

[30] Kao JH, Chen PJ, Lai MY, Chen DS. Basal core promoter mutations of hepatitis B virus increase the risk of hepatocellular carcinoma in hepatitis B carriers. Gastroenterology 2003;124(2) 327-334.

[31] Chan HLY, Hussain M, Lok ASF. Different hepatitis B virus genotypes are associated with different mutations in the core promoter and precore regions during Hepatitis B e antigen sero-conversion. Hepatology 1999;29(3) 976-984.

[32] Chan HLY, Leung NWY, Hussain M, Wong ML, Lok AS. Hepatitis B e antigen-negative chronic hepatitis B in Hong Kong. Hepatology 2000;31(3) 763-768.

[33] Fan ST, Lo CM, Poon RT, Yeung C, Liu CL, Yuen WK, Lam CM, Ng KK, Chan SC. Continuous improvement of survival outcomes of resection of hepatocellular carcinoma: a 20-year experience. Annals of Surgery 2011;253(4) 745-58.

[34] Chong CC, Lee KF, Ip PC, Wong JS, Cheung SY, Wong J, Ho SC, Lai PB. Pre-operative predictors of post-hepatectomy recurrence of hepatocellular carcinoma: can we predict earlier? Surgeon 2012;10(5) 260-6.

[35] Kudo M. Adjuvant therapy after curative treatment for hepatocellular carcinoma. Oncology 2011;81(Suppl 1) 50-55.

[36] Wong GLH, Wong VWS, Tan GM, Ip KI, Lai WK, Li YW, Mak MS, Lai PB, Sung JJ, Chan HL. Surveillance programme for hepatocellular carcinoma improves the survival of patients with chronic viral hepatitis. Liver International 2008;28(1) 79-87.

[37] Wu JC, Huang YH, Chau GY, Su CW, Lai CR, Lee PC, Huo TI, Sheen IJ, Lee SD, Lui WY. Risk factors for early and late recurrence in hepatitis B-related hepatocellular carcinoma. Journal of Hepatology 2009;51(5) 890-897.

[38] Sherman M. Recurrence of hepatocellular carcinoma. New England Journal of Medicine 2008;359(19) 2045-2047.

[39] Liao KF, Lai SW, Lin CY, Huang CH, Lin YY. Risk factors of recurrence after curative resection of hepatocellular carcinoma in Taiwan. The American journal of the medical sciences 2011;341(4) 301-304.

[40] Hung IFN, Poon RTP, Lai CL, Fung J, Fan ST and Yuen MF. Recurrence of hepatitis b-related hepatocellular carcinoma is associated with high viral load at the time of resection. American Journal of Gastroenterology 2008;103(7) 1663–1673.

[41] Huang Y, Wang Z, An S, Zhou B, Zhou Y, Chan HLY, Hou J. Role of hepatitis B virus genotypes and quantitative HBV DNA in metastasis and recurrence of hepatocellular carcinoma. Journal of Medical Virology 2008;80(4) 591-597.

[42] Cheung YS, Chan HLY, Wong J, Lee KF, Poon TC, Wong N, Lai PB. Elevated perioperative transaminase level predicts intrahepatic recurrence in hepatitis B-related hepatocellular carcinoma after curative hepatectomy. Asian Journal of Surgery 2008;31(2) 41-49.

[43] Iloeje UH, Yang HI, Su J, Jen CL, You CL, and Chen CJ. Predicting cirrhosis risk based on the level of circulating hepatitis B viral load. Gastroenterology 2006;130(3) 678–686.

[44] Liaw YF, Kao JH, Piratvisuth T et al. Asian-Pacific consensus statement on the management of chronic hepatitis B: a 2012 update. Hepatology International 2012.

[45] Matsumoto A, Tanaka E, Rokuhara A, Kiyosawa K, Kumada H, Omata M, Okita K, Hayashi N, Okanoue T, Iino S, Tanikawa K; the Inuyama Hepatitis Study Group. Efficacy of lamivudine for preventing hepatocellular carcinoma in chronic hepatitis B: A multicenter retrospective study of 2795 patients. Hepatology Research 2005;32(3) 173-184.

[46] Sung JJY, Tsoi KKF, Wong VWS, Li KC, Chan HLY. Meta-analysis: treatment of hepatitis B infection reduces risk of hepatocellular carcinoma. Alimentimentary Pharmacology and Therapeutics 2008;28(9) 1067–1077.

[47] Lok AS, McMahon BJ. Chronic hepatitis B. Hepatology 2007;45(2) 507-539.

[48] Wong GLH, Chan HLY. Predictors of treatment response in chronic hepatitis B. Drugs 2009;69(16) 2167-2177.

[49] Wong GLH. How does hepatitis B virus infection react to hepatocellular carcinoma treatment? Journal of Gastroenterology and Hepatology 2012;27(1) 1-2.

[50] Jang JW, Choi JY, Bae SH, Kim CW, Yoon SK, Cho SH, Yang JM, Ahn BM, Lee CD, Lee YS, Chung KW, Sun HS. Transarterial chemo-lipiodolization can reactivate hepatitis B virus replication in patients with hepatocellular carcinoma. Journal of Hepatology 2004;41(3) 427-435.

[51] Park JW, Park KW, Cho SH, Park HS, Lee WJ, Lee DH, Kim CM. Risk of hepatitis B exacerbation is low after transcatheter arterial chemoembolization therapy for patients with HBV-related hepatocellular carcinoma: report of a prospective study. American Journal of Gastroenterology 2005;100(10):2194-2200.

[52] Jang JW, Kwon JH, You CR, Kim JD, Woo HY, Bae SH, Choi JY, Yoon SK, Chung KW. Risk of HBV reactivation according to viral status and treatment intensity in patients with hepatocellular carcinoma. Antiviral Therapy 2011;16(7) 9699-9677.

[53] Huang L, Li J, Lau WY, Yan J, Zhou F, Liu C, Zhang X, Shen J, Wu M, Yan Y. Perioperative reactivation of hepatitis B virus replication in patients undergoing partial hepatectomy for hepatocellular carcinoma. Journal of Gastroenterology and Hepatology 2012;27(1) 158-164.

[54] Chen CJ, Yang HI. Natural history of chronic hepatitis B REVEALed. Journal of Gastroenterology and Hepatology 2011;26(4) 628-638.

[55] Thia TJK, Lui HF, Ooi LL, Chung YF, Chow PK, Cheow PC, Tan YM, Chow WC. A study into the risk of exacerbation of chronic hepatitis B after liver resection for hepatocellular carcinoma. Journal of Gastrointestinal Surgery 2007; 11(5) 612–618.

[56] Jang JW, Choi JY, Bae SH, Yoon SK, Chang UI, Kim CW, Cho SH, Han JY, Lee YS. A randomized controlled study of preemptive lamivudine in patients receiving transarterial chemo-lipiodolization. Hepatology 2006;43(2) 233-2340.

[57] Kim BK, Park JY, Kim do Y, Kim JK, Kim KS, Choi JS, Moon BS, Han KH, Chon CY, Moon YM, Ahn SH. Persistent hepatitis B viral replication affects recurrence of hepatocellular carcinoma after curative resection. Liver International 2008;28(3):393-401.

[58] Li N, Lai EC, Shi J, Guo WX, Xue J, Huang B, Lau WY, Wu MC, Cheng SQ. A comparative study of antiviral therapy after resection of hepatocellular carcinoma in the immune-active phase of hepatitis B virus infection. Annals of Surgical Oncology 2010; 17(1) 179–185.

[59] Kuzuya T, Katano Y, Kumada T, Toyoda H, Nakano I, Hirooka Y, Itoh A, Ishigami M, Hayashi K, Honda T, Goto H. Efficacy of antiviral therapy with lamivudine after initial treatment for hepatitis B virus-related hepatocellular carcinoma. Journal of Gastroenterology and Hepatology 2007; 22(11) 1929-1935.

[60] Miao RY, Zhao HT, Yang HY Mao YL, Lu X, Zhao Y, Liu CN, Zhong SX, Sang XT, Huang JF. Postoperative adjuvant antiviral therapy for hepatitis B/C virus-related hepatocellular carcinoma: a meta-analysis. World Journal of Gastroenterology 2010;16(23) 2931–2942.

[61] Wong JSW, Wong GLH, Tsoi KKF, Wong VW, Cheung SY, Chong CN, Wong J, Lee KF, Lai PB, Chan HL. Meta-analysis: the efficacy of anti-viral therapy in prevention of recurrence after curative treatment of chronic hepatitis B-related hepatocellular carcinoma. Alimentary Pharmacology and Therapeutics 2011;33(10) 1104-1112.

[62] Breitenstein S, Dimitroulis D, Petrowsky H, Puhan MA, Müllhaupt B, Clavien PA. Systematic review and meta-analysis of interferon after curative treatment of hepatocellular carcinoma in patients with viral hepatitis. British Journal of Surgery 2009;96(9) 975-981.

[63] Lau WY, Lai EC, Lau SH. The current role of neoadjuvant/ adjuvant/ chemoprevention therapy in partial hepatectomy for hepatocellular carcinoma: a systematic review. Hepatobiliary and Pancreatic Diseases International 2009;8(2) 124-133.

[64] Nevens F, Goubau P, Van Eyken P, Desmyter J, Desmet V, Fevery J. Treatment of decompensated viral hepatitis B-induced cirrhosis with low doses of interferon alpha. Liver 1993 13(1) 15-19.

[65] Liaw YF, Leung NW, Chang TT Guan R, Tai DI, Ng KY, Chien RN, Dent J, Roman L, Edmundson S, Lai CL. Effects of extended lamivudine therapy in Asian patients with chronic hepatitis B. Asia Hepatitis Lamivudine Study Group. Gastroenterology 2000;119(1) 172–180.

[66] Villeneuve JP, Condreay LD, Willems B, Pomier-Layrargues G, Fenyves D, Bilodeau M, Leduc R, Peltekian K, Wong F, Margulies M, Heathcote EJ. Lamivudine treatment for decompensated cirrhosis resulting from chronic hepatitis B. Hepatology 2000;31(1)207–210.

[67] Gane EJ, Chan HL, Ghoudhuri G, et al. Treatment of decompensated HBV-cirrhosis: results from 2-years randomized trial with telbivudine or lamivudine. Journal of Hepatology 2010;52(Suppl. 1) S4.

[68] Schwartz JD, Schwartz M, Mandeli J, Sung M. Neoadjuvant and adjuvant therapy for resectable hepatocellular carcinoma: review of the randomised clinical trials. Lancet Oncology 2002;3(10) 593–603.

[69] Kubo S, Tanaka H, Takemura S, Yamamoto S, Hai S, Ichikawa T, Kodai S, Shinkawa H, Sakaguchi H, Tamori A, Habu D, Nishiguchi S. Effects of lamivudine on outcome after liver resection for hepatocellular carcinoma in patients with active replication of hepatitis B virus. Hepatology Research 2007;37(2) 94–100.

[70] Koda M, Nagahara T, Matono T, Sugihara T, Mandai M, Ueki M, Ohyama K, Hosho K, Okano J, Kishimoto Y, Kono M, Maruyama S, Murawaki Y. Nucleotide analogs for patients with HBV-related hepatocellular carcinoma increase the survival rate through improved liver function. Internal Medicine 2009;48(1) 11–17.

[71] Lok AS, McMahon BJ. Chronic hepatitis B: update 2009. Hepatology 2009; 50(3) 661–662.

[72] Liaw YF, Leung N, Kao JH, Piratvisuth T, Gane E, Han KH, Guan R, Lau GK, Locarnini S; Chronic Hepatitis B Guideline Working Party of the Asian-Pacific Association for the Study of the Liver.. Asian-Pacific consensus statement on the management of chronic hepatitis B: a 2008 update. Hepatology International 2008;2(3) 263–283.

[73] European Association For The Study Of The Liver. EASL Clinical Practice Guidelines: management of chronic hepatitis B. Journal of Hepatology 2009;50(2) 227–242.

[74] Lui YYN, Tsoi KKF, Wong VWS, Kao JH, Hou JL, Teo EK, Mohamed R, Piratvisuth T, Han KH, Mihm U, Wong GL, Chan HL. Cost-effectiveness analysis of roadmap

models in chronic hepatitis B using tenofovir as the rescue therapy. Antiviral Theraoy 2010; 15(2) 145–155.

[75] Yuen MF, Yuan HJ, Wong DKH, Yuen JC, Wong WM, Chan AO, Wong BC, Lai KC, Lai CL. Prognostic determinants for chronic hepatitis B in Asians: therapeutic implications. Gut 2005;54(11) 1610–1614.

[76] Lai M and Liaw YF. Chronic hepatitis B: past, present, and future. Clinics in Liver Disease 2010;14(3) 531–546.

[77] Ikeda K, Arase Y, Kobayashi M, Saitoh S, Someya T, Hosaka T, Suzuki Y, Suzuki F, Tsubota A, Akuta N, Kumada H. Significance of multicentric cancer recurrence after potentially curative ablation of hepatocellular carcinoma: a long-term cohort study of 892 patients with viral cirrhosis. Journal of Gastroenterology 2003;38(9) 865–876.

Chapter 4

Immunotherapy for Hepatocellular Carcinoma: Current Status and Future Perspectives

Yu Sawada, Kazuya Ofuji, Mayuko Sakai and Tetsuya Nakatsura

Additional information is available at the end of the chapter

http://dx.doi.org/10.5772/54594

1. Introduction

For most patients with advanced hepatocellular carcinoma (HCC), surgery with curative intent or a locally ablative technique, such as percutaneous ethanol injection or radiofrequency ablation, are no longer available [1]. Patients can now be treated using transarterial chemoembolization (TACE) or systemic chemotherapy. Several chemotherapeutic drugs have been developed and tested. The anti-tumor effect of these treatments is limited and adverse reactions are not tolerated in advanced HCC patients with liver cirrhosis, which affects drug metabolism and toxicity [1-3]. Thus far, sorafenib, a multi-targeted tyrosine kinase inhibitor, is the only drug that has been shown to significantly prolong survival (by nearly 3 months) in patients with advanced HCC [4, 5]. However, the incidence of adverse drug reactions is high, particularly in elderly patients, and no second-line treatment has been established for patients who have failed sorafenib treatment [6]. Thus, new treatment modalities are urgently required to prolong survival in patients with advanced HCC while minimizing the risk of adverse reactions.

The 5-year recurrence rate of HCC exceeds 70% after surgery or radiofrequency ablation due to a high risk of metastasis and development of *de novo* HCC in a cirrhotic liver [7,8]. The relapse-free survival rate was reported to be improved by adjuvant therapy with vitamin K2 [9], retinoid [10], or interferon [11-13]. These reports have not as yet been validated, and these treatments to prevent relapse are not widely adopted. In recent years, clinical trials of sorafenib have been conducted to explore its role in adjuvant therapy [14]. However, these data are unpublished and a standard adjuvant therapy has not been established. Establishment of an effective preventative method, such as vaccination to prevent the occurrence and recurrence of HCC, is also required.

Immunotherapy is a potentially attractive option for HCC, and induction of tumor-specific reactions without autoimmunity is the ideal strategy. Many fundamental studies have demonstrated that tumor cells can be targeted by various immune effector mechanisms. Previous immunotherapeutic clinical trials in patients with advanced HCC have shown mainly its feasibility and safety [15,16]. However, no non-randomized phase I or II studies have demonstrated the efficacy of immunotherapy for advanced HCC [16]. Conversely, several randomized controlled trials, in adjuvant settings, have shown its ability to reduce the risk of cancer recurrence [17-19].

This chapter aims to overview current knowledge concerning the progress of immunotherapy for HCC, including preclinical data and clinical trials, and to introduce our fundamental studies and clinical trials of the glypican-3 (GPC3)-derived peptide vaccine.

2. Concepts of antitumor immunity

The aim of immunotherapy against cancer is to provide clinical benefit by activating the immune system. Various immunotherapy strategies have been investigated in preclinical and clinical trials to accomplish this purpose. The diversity of strategies is due to the fact that tumor cells can be targeted by various immune effector mechanisms, such as lymphokine-activated killer (LAK) cells, natural killer (NK) cells, T cells, dendritic cells, cytokine therapy, and antibody treatment. The induction of long-lasting tumor-specific reactions without autoimmunity is the ideal immunotherapeutic strategy and has been investigated extensively, particularly for melanoma and renal cell carcinoma. Rosenberg reported a dramatic clinical effect of adoptive cell therapy (ACT) using autologous tumor-infiltrating lymphocytes (TILs) against metastatic melanoma [20]. Also, TILs derived from HCC, after *ex vivo* expansion with interleukin-2 (IL-2), can lyse autologous tumors [21]. Furthermore, patients with HCC infiltrated by lymphocytes demonstrate a better prognosis after resection [22]. Thus the immune system, activated in various ways, can recognize and eliminate cancer cells, including HCC, although these cells may develop various mechanisms of escape from this action (Figure 1).

2.1. HCC antigenic targets

Tumor-specific antigens are the principal targets of immunotherapy, including in cancer vaccines, in ACT, and as monoclonal antibodies (mAbs). Thus, identification of appropriate tumor-specific antigens is the first and important step for progress of immunotherapy. Tumor-specific CD8+ T cells are considered to be critical for cancer control. They recognize 8- to 11-amino acid peptides that are derived from intracellular proteins called tumor antigens, which are presented in association with HLA class I complexes. Various tumor antigens and their cytotoxic T lymphocyte (CTL) epitopes have been identified and investigated in HCC.

Alpha-fetoprotein (AFP) is a representative HCC tumor-specific antigen. The onco-fetal antigen AFP, considered an ideal serological marker, is expressed in 50–80% of HCC. Various human leukocyte antigen (HLA)-A2- or HLA-A24-restricted AFP-specific epitopes have been identified. AFP has been shown to be an effective tumor rejection antigen in murine HCC [23]. Additionally, an AFP-derived peptide vaccine has been demonstrated to induce antigen-specific CD8 T-cell response in HCC patients [24]. In HCC, AFP is the most commonly investigated antigen, and several AFP-based immunotherapy regimens have been reported; however, no dramatic clinical benefit was observed [24,25].

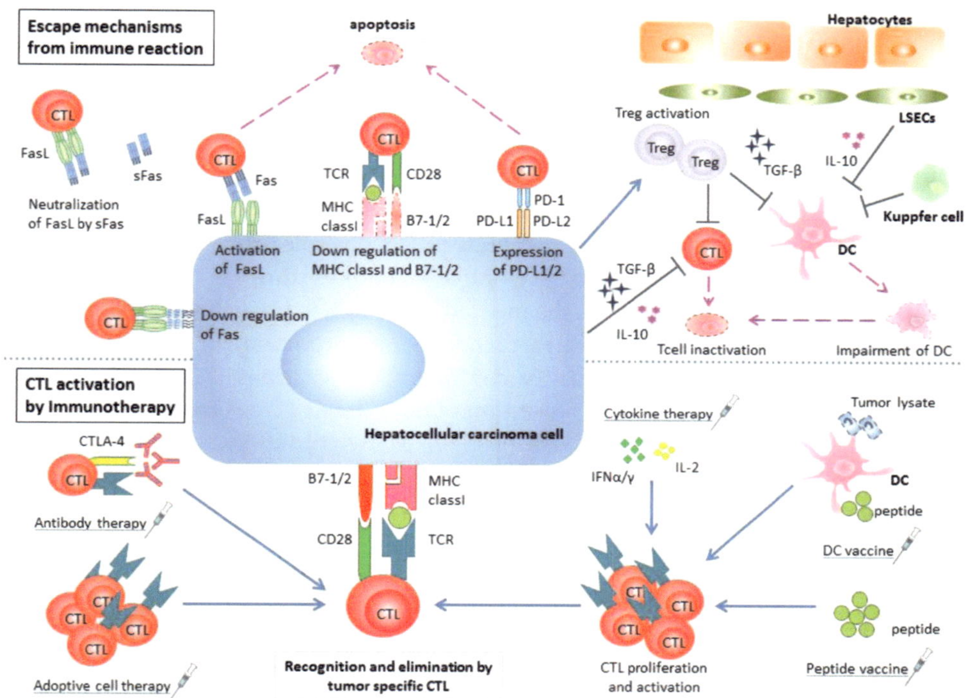

Figure 1. Immunotherapy against hepatocellular carcinoma cells. A number of strategies exist for induction of antitumor immunity against hepatocellular carcinoma cells. Tumor-specific cytotoxic T lymphocytes (CTLs) activated by various immunotherapies are capable of recognizing and eliminating cancer cells. However, tumor cells have developed various mechanisms of escape from antitumor reactions. Increased comprehension of the mechanisms underlying the immune-privileged status of the liver and escape of tumors from immune reactions will increase the efficacy of immunotherapy.

MAGE and NY-ESO-1, cancer testis antigens, are also expressed in HCC tumors. Normally, tumor testis antigens are expressed only in the testis and/or ovary. Additionally, major histocompatibility complex (MHC) class I antigens are not expressed on germ cells; thus, they are considered promising cancer vaccine candidate antigens. MAGE-A was initially identified in melanoma [26], and later found to be expressed in another cancers, including HCC [27], lung cancer, breast cancer, oral squamous cell carcinoma, and esophageal carcinoma. Some CTL epitopes of the MAGE family have been identified in HCC.

NY-ESO-1 was identified in a patient with squamous cell carcinoma of the esophagus [28]. NY-ESO-1 is expressed in various cancers, including melanoma, lung cancer, ovarian cancer, breast cancer, and HCC. NY-ESO-1 is characterized by its high immunogenicity and is considered a good target molecule for antigen-specific immunotherapy.

GPC3, a heparan sulfate proteoglycan, was previously reported to be overexpressed in HCC [29]. The carcinoembryonic antigen GPC3 plays an important role in cell growth and differentiation and is considered an ideal tumor antigen for immunotherapy; this antigen is discussed further below.

2.2. Dendritic cells

Dendritic cells (DCs) are the most potent antigen-presenting cells (APCs), and are composed of multiple subsets, primarily conventional and plasmacytoid DCs [30]. DCs play an important role in both induction of antitumor immunity and tolerance. The DC vaccine, loaded with tumor-specific antigens, is considered to stimulate a specific T-cell response. Several methods of antigen loading to DCs exist, including peptide pulsing, whole protein loading, and genetic engineering. DC-based immunotherapy is highly complex due to the various possible strategies, such as the DC subset used, the method of antigen loading, and the administration route (subcutaneous, intravenous, intralymph node, or intratumoral). Figdor *et al.* provided a roadmap for standardization and quality control of DC vaccines [31]. In HCC patients, enhanced NK-cell activation and decreased regulatory T-cell (Treg) frequencies have been identified after administration of DC vaccines [32]. Many studies suggested that DC-based immunotherapies for HCC could stimulate a tumor-specific T-cell response leading to clinical benefit without any significant toxicity.

2.3. Cytokine therapy and immunostimulatory mAbs

The effects of immunostimulatory cytokines in HCC have been investigated, such as interferon-alpha (IFN-α), interferon-gamma (IFN-γ), and interleukin (IL)-2. These elicit a nonspecific immune response.

As an antiviral agent, IFN-α is often used against hepatitis B or hepatitis C virus infection to prevent progression to HCC. IFN-α, by enhancing cytotoxicity, tumor antigen presentation, proliferation of lymphocytes, and anti-angiogenesis, induces an antitumor response [33,34]. IFN-α treatment for HCC has been reported to have some clinical efficacy, likely by preventing or delaying tumor recurrence after surgical resection or ablation [35,36]. IFN-α has been tested in combination with chemotherapy for advanced HCC [37,38]. Adverse side effects are an important issue in IFN-based therapy, particularly for patients with severe liver injury.

IFN-γ, which improves antigen presentation and lymphocyte activation, has also been used for advanced HCC in combination with chemotherapy [39] or granulocyte-macrophage colony stimulating factor (GM-CSF) [40]. However, no clinical response was identified.

IL-2, one of the most immunostimulatory cytokines, plays an important role in regulation of immune activation and homeostasis. IL-2 has various effects on immune cells, such as CD4+ T cells, CD8+ T cells, B cells and NK cells [41]. The effect of IL-2 in various cancers has been investigated, particularly melanoma and renal cell carcinoma. In HCC, several IL-2 treatment regimens have been reported, with or without combination therapy [42,43].

In 1975, the procedure for generation of hybridomas was published [44]. Subsequently, mAbs have been developed as diagnostic and therapeutic agents. In the field of cancer therapy, mAbs that activate the immune system against tumor cells, inhibit cancer cell-intrinsic signaling pathways, bring toxins close to cancer cells, or interfere with the tumor-stroma interaction have been developed [45].

Several anti-costimulatory molecule antibodies that activate the immune response have been investigated. For example, a mAb against the costimulatory molecule CD28, the receptor of the family of B7 antigens, has been investigated. For T-cell activation, both binding of the T-cell receptor to antigen and costimulatory signaling by CD28 are needed [46]. Some CD28 mAbs called 'superagonists' can stimulate and expand T cells in the absence of T cell antigen receptor (TCR) ligation [47]. In a phase I trial of an anti-CD28 mAb, severe toxicity was observed [48].

The CTL-associated antigen 4 (CTLA-4), a homolog of CD28, is an inhibitory receptor for B7 [49] that functions as an immune check point and downregulates T-cell activation pathways by competing with CD28 for binding to B7 [50,51]. The clinical benefit of ipilimumab, anti CTLA-4 mAb, against advanced melanoma has been reported [52,53]; its use has been approved by the United States Food and Drug Administration.

2.4. Escape mechanisms from immune reactions

As mentioned above, cancer cells can be targeted by various immunotherapeutic strategies. However, cancer cells possess mechanisms of escape from the immune response. Additionally, the liver is considered an immune-privileged organ. The liver contains at least three types of APCs; *i.e.*, Kupffer cells (KCs), liver sinusoidal endothelial cells (LSECs), and dendritic cells, which might be associated with its immune-privileged status [54]. KCs and LSECs constitutively express the anti-inflammatory cytokines IL-10 and transforming growth factor beta (TGF-β) [55,56]. These immunosuppressive cytokines may play a role in immune privilege by influencing T-cell differentiation and suppressing APC maturation. Furthermore, hepatic stellate cells (also known as Ito cells), a liver-specific cell population that is found between the sinusoids and hepatocytes, promote hepatic inflammation. Hepatic stellate cells express TGF-β only after chronic liver injury [57,58].

2.4.1. Impairment of DC function

One of the mechanisms of tumor escape from the immune response is impairment of DC function. In cancer patients, inadequate DC function has been suggested to be related to non-responsiveness to antitumor immunity [59]. Immunosuppressive factors that inhibit DC maturation are released from tumors. For instance, human cancer cells release vascular endothelial growth factor (VEGF), which inhibits the maturation of DCs [60]. Other cytokines derived from tumors, such as IL-6 [61] and IL-10 [62], also influence the function of DCs.

Additionally, DCs have reduced function in cancers, including HCC, in that they cannot stimulate T cells [63,64].

2.4.2. Antigen presentation

It is clear that the level of MHC class I expression on the cell surface is crucial for CD8+ T cell cytotoxicity against target cells. Decreased or absent MHC class I expression, which facilitates tumor escape from immune surveillance, has been reported in various tumors. Additionally, in HCC, HLA class I expression on tumor cells may be down-regulated [65,66]. However, strong HLA class I expression in HCC has also been reported [67]. Thus, the level of MHC class I expression in HCC is unclear. Furthermore, expression of the co-stimulatory molecules B7-1 and B7-2 is reduced in HCC [66]. Such down-regulation causes impairment of tumor-antigen processing and presentation.

2.4.3. Inhibitory molecules

Another escape mechanism involves over- or reduced expression of molecules associated with cell death, such as Fas/FasL, PD-1/PD-L1, CTLA-4, and Decoy receptor 3. Fas is a cell-surface protein that belongs to the family of tumor necrosis factor (TNF) receptors [68]. Fas ligand (FasL) is a type II membrane protein that binds to Fas [69]. Cross-linking of Fas with FasL induces apoptosis of Fas-bearing cells [70]. FasL is found in immune-privileged sites, such as the testis and eye [71,72]. HCC tissues have been reported to express Fas weakly and at a low frequency [73]. Additionally, elevated soluble Fas (sFas) levels in HCC patients have been reported [74]. Loss of cell-surface Fas in HCC and neutralization of FasL by sFas might be involved in tumor cell immune escape [75].

PD-L1 is member of the B7 family that can interact with programmed death-1 (PD-1). Its receptor, PD-1, is expressed on activated T and B cells and elicits inhibitory signals [76]. PD-L1 is expressed on dendritic cells, macrophages, and parenchymal cells, as well as various human cancer cells. The objective response of the PD-1 antibody against non-small cell lung cancer, melanoma, or renal cell cancer has been suggested to be related to PD-L1 expression on tumor cells [77]. In HCC, PD-1 expression is upregulated on effector-phase CD8+ T cells, particularly in tumor-infiltrating CD8+ T cells [78]. High expression of PD-1 on T cells both in TILs and peripheral blood mononuclear cells (PBMCs) is correlated with a poor prognosis in HCC patients after surgical resection [78]. Additionally, PD-L1 expression on Kupffer cells (KC) has been shown to be increased in tumor tissues in patients with HCC, and is correlated with poor survival [79]. These suggest that effector phase T-cell inhibition is associated with tumor survival.

Decoy receptor 3 (DcR3), a member of the TNF receptor superfamily, might also be involved in immune escape. DcR3 inhibits FasL-induced apoptosis by binding to its ligand Fas. Additionally, DcR3 overexpression in HCC has been reported [80,81].

2.4.4. Regulatory T cells

CD4+CD25+ regulatory T cells (Tregs) can suppress other immune cells and are critical mediators of self-tolerance. Tregs also suppress the immune response against cancer cells.

High numbers of Tregs were detected in peripheral blood and TILs in HCC patients [82, 83]. CD4+CD25+FoxP3+ Tregs could impair the cytotoxic function of tumor-infiltrating CD8+ T cells [84]. Levels of the immunosuppressive cytokine IL-10 are increased in HCC patients, a finding that is related to Treg induction [85]. Thus, CD4+CD25+ Tregs may play an important role in regulating the immune response against HCC.

The goal of immunotherapy against human cancers, including HCC, is to impact target tumor cells without influencing normal cell function. Comprehension of the mechanisms of the immune-privileged status of the liver and escape of tumors from immune reactions will increase the efficacy of immunotherapy.

3. Clinical trials

Clinical trials of immunotherapy to enhance anti-tumor responses in patients with advanced HCC, or to reduce the risk of recurrence after curative treatment have been conducted (Table 1).

Author	Country	Year	Indication	Immunotherapy	n	Clinical result	Reference
Takayama T, et al.	Japan	2000	Adjuvant (resection)	RCT: activated autologous lymphocyte vs. no treatment	76 and 74	Significantly longer recurrence-free survival after transfer of activated lymphocytes (p=0.008)	[17]
Llovet JM, et al.	Spain	2000	Advanced HCC	RCT: IFN-α2b vs. no treatment	30 and 28	RR: 2/30 (7%), DCR: NA No significant difference in RR and survival	[156]
Ikeda K, et al.	Japan	2000	Adjuvant (resection or ethanol injection)	RCT: IFN-β vs. no treatment	10 and 10	Significantly longer recurrence-free survival after IFN-β therapy (p=0.0004	[11]
Kubo S, et al.	Japan	2001	Adjuvant (resection)	RCT: IFN-α vs. no treatment	15 and 15	Significantly longer recurrence-free survival after IFN-α therapy (p=0.037)	[12]
Reinisch W, et al.	Austria	2002	Advanced HCC	GM-CSF + IFN-γ	15	RR: 1/15 (7%), DCR: 10/15 (67%) MST: 5.5 months	[40]
Palmieri G, et al.	Italy	2002	Advanced HCC	Low dose IL-2	18	RR: 3/18 (17%), DCR: 16/18 (89%) MST: 24.5 months	[42]

Author	Country	Year	Indication	Immunotherapy	n	Clinical result	Reference
Ladhams A, et al.	Australia	2002	Advanced HCC	Dendritic cell pulsed with autologous tumor	2	Slowing in the rate of tumor growth in one of two patients	[157]
Sakon M, et al.	Japan	2002	Advanced HCC	5-FU + IFN-α	11	RR: 8/11 (73%), DCR: 9/11 (82%) MST: NA	[158]
Iwashita, et al.	Japan	2003	Advanced HCC	Dendritic cell pulsed with autologous tumor	10 (8 HCC)	RR: 0/8 (0%), DCR 6/8 (75%) MST: NA	[114]
Patt YZ, et al.	USA	2003	Advanced HCC	5-FU + IFN-α2b	43	RR: 9/36 (25%), DCR 22/36 (61%) MST: 19.5 months	[37]
Stift A, et al.	Austria	2003	Advanced HCC	Dendritic cell pulsed with autologous tumor	20 (2 HCC)	RR: NA, DCR: NA MST: 10.5 months Constant remaining of AFP over a period of 6 months in one of two patients	[159]
Feun LG, et al.	USA	2003	Advanced HCC	Doxorubicin + 5-FU + IFN-α2b	30	RR: 2/30 (7%), DCR: 3/30 (10%) MST: 3 months	[160]
Komorizono Y, et al.	Japan	2003	Advanced HCC	Cisplatin + 5-FU + IFN-α	6	RR: 2/6 (33%), DCR 3/6 (50%) MST: NA	[38]
Butterfield, et al.	USA	2003	Advanced HCC	AFP peptide vaccination	6	RR: 0/6 (0%), DCR 0/6 (0%) MST: 8 months	[24]
Shiratori Y, et al.	Japan	2003	adjuvant (ethanol injection)	RCT: IFN-α vs. no treatment	49 and 25	Longer recurrence-free and overall survival after IFN-α therapy (p-value not shown)	[13]
Kuang M, et al.	China	2004	Adjuvant	RCT: autologous formalin-fixed tumor vaccine vs. no treatment	18 and 21	Significantly longer recurrence-free survival after vaccination (p=0.003)	[18]
Shi M, et al	China	2004	Advanced and early HCC	Cytokine induced killer cell	13	RR: NA, DCR: NA MST: NA	[161]
Sangro B, et al.	Spain	2004	Advanced HCC	Intratumoral adenovirus encoding IL-12 genes	21 (8 HCC)	RR: 1/8 (13%), DCR 7/8 (88%) MST: NA	[162]

Author	Country	Year	Indication	Immunotherapy	n	Clinical result	Reference
Lee WC, et al.	Taiwan	2005	Advanced HCC	Dendritic cell pulsed with autologous tumor	31	RR: 4/31 (13%), DCR 21/31 (68%) MST: NA	[163]
Kumagai, et al.	Japan	2005	Advanced HCC	Intratumoral dendritic cell injection after ethanol injection	4	Feasibility study	[164]
Yin XY, et al.	China	2005	Advanced HCC	Cisplatin + doxorubicin + 5-FU + IFN-2α	26	RR: 4/26 (15%), DCR 13/26 (50%) MST: 6 months	[165]
Chi KH	Taiwan	2005	Advanced HCC	Local radiation + intratumoral DC injection	14	RR: 2/14 (14%), DCR 9/14 (64%) MST: 5.6 months	[113]
Mazzolini G, et al.	Spain	2005	Advanced HCC	Dendritic cell transfected with adenovirus encoding IL-12 gene	17 (8 HCC)	RR: 0/0 (0%), DCR: 2/8 (25%) MST: NA	[166]
Butterfield, et al.	USA	2006	Advanced HCC	Dendritic cell pulsed with AFP peptide	10	RR: 0/10 (0%), DCR 0/10 (0%) MST: 7.5 months	[25]
Nakamoto Y, et al.	Japan	2007	Advanced and early HCC	Non-RCT: TACE + dendritic cell vs. TACE alone	10 and 11	No significant difference in survival	[141]
Vitale FV, et al.	Italy	2007	Advanced HCC	5-FU + IFN-α2b	9	RR: 3/9 (33%), DCR 4/9 (44%) MST: 11.5 months	[167]
Weng DS, et al.	China	2008	Adjuvant (TACE and RFA)	RCT: cytokine induced killer cell vs. no treatment	45 and 40	Significantly longer recurrence-free survival after immunotherapy (p=0.01)	[168]
Hui D, et al.	China	2009	Adjuvant (resection)	RCT: cytokine induced killer cell 3 courses vs. 6 courses vs. no treatment	41, 43 and 43	Significantly longer recurrence-free survival after immunotherapy (p=0.001 and 0.004)	[169]
Palmer DH, et al.	UK	2009	Advanced HCC	Dendritic cell pulsed with liver tumor cell line lysate (HepG2)	35	RR: 1/25 (4%), DCR 7/25 (28%) MST: 5.6 months	[170]
Olioso P, et al.	Italy	2009	Advanced HCC	Cytokine induced killer cell + IFN-α	12 (1 HCC)	Complete response Survival time: 33 months (alive)	[171]

Author	Country	Year	Indication	Immunotherapy	n	Clinical result	Reference
Hao MZ, et al.	China	2010	Advanced HCC	Non-RCT: TACE + cytokine induced killer cell vs. TACE alone	72 and 74	Significantly longer survival after combination therapy ($p<0.001$)	[172]
Greten TF, et al	Germany	2010	Advanced HCC	a telomerase peptide vaccine in combinatuon with a low dose cyclophosphamide	40	RR: 0/40 (0%), DCR 17/37 (45.9%) MST: 9.8 months	[139]
Ma H, et al.	China	2010	Adjuvant (RFA)	RFA and autologous RetroNectin activated killer cells	7	During a seven-month follow-up, no severe adverse events, recurrences or deaths	[173]
Zhou P, et al.	China	2011	HCC with hepatitis B(PMWA)	Immature DCs, cytokine-induced killer cells (CIK), cytotoxic T lymphocytes (CTL) and tumor lysate-pulsed DC	10	This phase I study revealed this therapy was safe and increased the percentage of effector cells.	[174]
Sawada Y, et al.	Japan	2012	Advanced HCC	GPC3-derived peptide vaccine	33	RR: 1/33 (3%), DCR 20/33 (60.6%) MST: 9.0 months OS was significantly longer in patients with high GPC3-specific CTL frequencies	[120]

HCC; hepatocellular carcinoma, LAK; lymphokine-activated killer cell, IL; interleukin, RR; response rate, DCR; disease control rate, MST; median survival time, IFN; interferon, NA; not assessed, RCT; randomised control trial, CTL; cytotoxic T lymphocyte, TIL; tumor-infiltrating lymphocyte, TACE; transcatheter arterial chemoembolization, GM-CSF; granulocyte macrophage colony-stimulating factor, RFA; radiofrequency ablation therapy, PMWA; percutaneous microwave ablation

Table 1. Immunotherapeutic clinical trials in HCC after 2000

3.1. Cytokine therapy

3.1.1. IFN-α

IFN-α has direct antitumor effects on tumor cells, including induction of lymphocytes, macrophage cytotoxic activities, and anti-angiogenesis.

A number of trials have evaluated the clinical efficacy of IFN-α in HCC. Lai *et al.* reported that IFN-α was useful in patients with inoperable HCC, in terms of both prolonging survival and inducing tumor regression [86]. However, a high IFN-α dose can cause toxicity [12]; thus, systemic administration of IFN-α [12] or IFN-β [11] should be considered

http://dx.doi.org/10.5772/54594

as supportive treatment after hepatectomy or tumor ablation, which may prevent or delay tumor recurrence. Combination therapy with IFN-α and chemotherapy was applied in advanced HCC patients; however, no benefit was identified other than tolerance of the therapy for cirrhotic patients [13].

3.1.2. IL-2

IL-2 is an immunostimulatory cytokine that is used singly or in combination with other treatments in patients with liver tumors. Systemic induction of IL-2 produces objective responses against HCC when administered alone [42] or in combination with melatonin [43] or lymphokine-activated killer (LAK) cells [87].

3.1.3. IFN-γ

Lygidakis *et al.* reported that combination therapy with hepatic transarterial locoregional chemotherapy and immunotherapy that included IFN-γ and IL-2 is a promising therapeutic approach for advanced HCC [39]. This highlights the effect of IFN-γ. Moreover, GM-CSF and IFN-γ were effective in selected advanced HCC patients [40].

Systemic IL-12 and TNF-α treatment has been reported to cause severe toxicity in other cancers. However, there is to our knowledge no report of their effect against primary or metastatic liver cancer.

Although cytokine treatment for HCC can have positive outcomes, toxic effects can result, including systemic vascular leak syndrome.

Cytokines, such as IL-7 and IL-15, may be reasonable adjuvants due to their vaccination and culture properties.

3.2. Gene transfer

Transfer of immunostimulatory cytokine genes has effects on immune tolerance against tumors. Clinical trials with gene transfer therapy have been evaluated. Presently, this procedure is a safe and represents a novel therapeutic approach.

There are two main approaches to transfer of genes: 1) direct injection of vectors expressing cytokines, chemokines, or costimulatory molecules into tumor lesions, or 2) use of tumor cells or DCs transduced *ex vivo* with vectors expressing cytokines or costimulatory molecules [88].

IL-12 is a potent cytokine that shows antitumor activity in some models [89,90]. Although the effect of IL-12 gene transfer for liver tumor treatment in animal models has been reported, its use in early clinical trials of cancer patients has shown no significant benefit [91].

Abnormally elevated levels of Th2 cytokines, such as IL-10, skews the immune response to favor tumor growth. Conversely, Lopez *et al.* showed that the combination of autologous inactivated tumor cells expressing IL-12 and IL-10 induced tumor remission in 50–70% of mice with large established colon or mammary tumors and spontaneous lung metastases, with consequent establishment of an antitumor immune memory [92]. Systemic injection of IL-2 in patients with metastatic renal carcinoma and melanoma showed a low efficacy and high toxicity. A phase I–II clinical trial of recombinant adenovirus encoding the IL-2 gene was performed in patients with advanced carcinoma. Only one patient showed a positive response in terms of tumor necrosis [93].

Molecules such as HLA-B7 are important for promotion of specific T-cell responses. Total or selective loss of MHS class I antigens has been reported in some malignancies [94,95]. Animal studies have demonstrated that injection of foreign MHC molecules can result in immunologic destruction of the tumor by eliciting a T-cell-dependent immune response not only to the foreign MHC protein, but also to previously unrecognized tumor-associated antigens. Rubin *et al*. showed that indirect intralesional gene transfer therapy of both HLA-B7 and β2-microglobulin for colorectal cancer (CRC) patients with hepatic metastasis had no serious toxicity and was feasible; however, details of any antitumor effect were not reported [96].

Oncolytic virotherapy is based on the ability of viral vectors to replicate selectively in cancer cells and thus exert a direct antitumor effect [97]. Adenovirus is one of the most common viral vectors [98]. dl1520 is a mutant oncolytic adenovirus [99]. Habib *et al*. reported that dl1520 gene therapy had no significant antitumor effect in HCC patients compared with percutaneous ethanol injection [100]. A phase I clinical trial of intratumoral administration of a first-generation adenoviral vector-encoding herpes simplex virus thymidine kinase (HSV-TK) gene (Ad.TK) to HCC patients was conducted. Treatment was well-tolerated and no dose-limiting toxicity occurred. Sixty percent of patients showed tumor stabilization and, importantly, two patients who received the highest dose showed signs of intratumoral necrosis using imaging procedures [101].

Additionally, Kottke *et al*. showed that, in mice, oncolytic virotherapy could lead to direct tumor cell lysis and could trigger innate immune-mediated attack on tumor vascularization when combined with antiangiogenic cancer therapy [102].

Transfer of cytokine genes and oncolytic viruses is currently under development and represents a promising new approach for treatment of human cancer. Recent technical advances in the genetic modification of oncolytic viruses have improved their tumor specificity. Clinical trials with oncolytic viruses demonstrate the safety and feasibility of this approach. Systemic administration of oncolytic viruses represents a novel approach to treatment of a range of tumors [103].

3.3. Effector cells and adoptive T-cell therapy

Several trials have evaluated the induction of various types of cytotoxic lymphocytes. One report compared adoptive chemoimmunotherapy with chemotherapy. Chemoimmunotherapy comprised arterial infusion of adriamycin, recombinant interleukin-2, and lymphokine-activated killer cells, whereas chemotherapy comprised administration of adriamycin alone. No significant difference between the two groups was found; thus adoptive chemoimmunotherapy was concluded to not be an ideal adjuvant protocol after hepatic resection [104].

The reason that LAK cells demonstrate no benefit may be their lack of tumor-antigen specificity. In contrast, TILs with anti-tumor activity are induced during the natural course of tumor growth. Thus, TILs have been shown to contain tumor antigen-specific T cells [20]. In one study, indium^{111}-labeled TILs activated by IL-2 and CD3 mAbs were injected via intrahepatic arteries in three patients with hepatic malignancies and their distribution was evaluated. TILs accumulated in the liver and persisted for at least 48 h after infusion. After intra-arterial chemoimmunotherapy that included TILs, two of three patients achieved a partial therapeutic response. This method may facilitate accumulation of TILs at tumor sites, likely augmenting the antitumor effects of adoptive immunotherapy [105].

In the largest randomized trial, 150 patients who had undergone curative resection for HCC received either IL-2 with anti-CD3-activated peripheral blood lymphocytes or underwent observation. Adoptive immunotherapy decreased the frequency of recurrence and prolonged the time to first recurrence compared with the control group. Additionally, the immunotherapy group demonstrated a significantly longer recurrence-free survival and disease-specific survival than the control group. However, overall survival did not differ significantly between groups, providing more objective support for the potential of immunotherapy [17].

Adoptive T-cell therapy includes passive transfer of antigen-reactive T cells to a tumor-bearing host to initiate tumor rejection. Based on animal models, effector T cells with tumor-specific reactivity are superior to non-specific effector T cells in terms of mediating tumor regression *in vivo* [106].

However, translation of these successful methods into patients is not yet feasible due to difficulties in generation of tumor antigen-specific T cells *ex vivo* [107]. In general, adoptive T-cell therapy is accomplished by harvesting cells from peripheral blood, tumor sites (TILs), or draining lymph nodes, and identifying tumor-associated antigens (TAAs). TAAs are ectopically expressed or overexpressed in tumor cells relative to normal tissues. One of the most important HCC TAAs is AFP. AFP-based immunotherapy has been applied in HCC. Grimm *et al.* immunized mice bearing m-AFP-expressing HCC using DNA expression vectors encoding mAFP. Some mice developed mAFP antibody responses, which were associated with a significant survival benefit. These data suggested that AFP has the potential to function as a tumor antigen, inducing CTLs and CD4+ T-cell-mediated regression of AFP-positive HCC [108].

Many other TAAs that are tumor-specific "cancer-testis" antigens in HCC (MAGE, GAGE, BAGE, NY-ESO, CTA, TSPY, FATE/Bj-HCC-2, and GPC3, among others) have been identified [109]. GPC3 is a specific immunomarker of HCC and induces effective antitumor immunity in mice [110]. Several antigens, such as CEA and CP1, are also known to be TAAs of CRC liver tumors [111].

3.4. APCs

A number of strategies utilize the immune-activating ability of professional APCs, particularly DCs. T-cell activation can result from DC cross presentation. Thus, mature DCs can induce antitumor immunity [112]. A phase I study of the safety and efficacy of direct injection of autologous immature DCs into tumors under radiotherapy was conducted. A decrease in the AFP level of greater than 50% was identified in three patients, and NK activity was enhanced [113].

Addition of tumor lysate or purified proteins to immature DCs improves their function as APC. Iwashita *et al*. used autologous DCs pulsed with tumor lysate (TL) and evaluated their safety and feasibility. Immunization with TL-pulsed DCs was well-tolerated and feasible. In one patient, one of two liver tumors showed necrotic changes and, in two patients, serum levels of tumor markers decreased after vaccination [114].

Morse *et al*. concluded that combination therapy with DCs pulsed with a CEA peptide and adjuvant cytokines (IFN-α and TNF-α) in patients with CEA-expressing malignancy showed no toxicity and was feasible [115]. Brat *et al*. showed that peptide-loaded DCs enhanced NK cell activation and decreased Treg frequencies in vaccinated HCC patients [32].

Thus, the potential of DCs to improve treatment of many cancers has been confirmed, and various strategies are now being developed.

3.5. Peptide vaccines

Douglas *et al*. showed that gp100 peptide vaccine and IL-2 combination therapy resulted in progression-free survival longer than IL-2 alone in patients with advanced melanoma [116]. The peptide vaccine was tolerated and yielded favorable immunologic responses, such as induction of peptide-specific CTLs or reduced Tregs [117,118].

Regarding HCC, the AFP-derived peptide vaccine induced antigen-specific CD8 T-cell responses; however, no dramatic clinical benefit was identified [24].

The GPC3-derived peptide vaccine can induce high-avidity CTLs capable of killing GPC3-expressing HCC cells [119]. A phase I trial of the GPC3-derived vaccine for advanced HCC indicated that the vaccine was well-tolerated and that peptide-specific CTLs could be a predictive marker of overall survival [120]. The GPC3 peptide vaccine is discussed further in the next section.

4. The GPC3-derived peptide vaccine: our fundamental sutdies and clinical trials

4.1. GPC3, an ideal tumor antigen

GPC3 is a member of the glypican family of heparan sulfate proteoglycans, which are attached to the cell surface via the glycosylphosphatidylinositol (GPI) anchor [121]. GPC3 forms a complex with Wnt molecules and promotes the growth of HCC by stimulating canonical Wnt signaling [122]. We reported that GPC3 was specifically overexpressed in human HCC based on cDNA microarray data [29]. We reported that GPC3 is an ideal tumor antigen for immunotherapy in mouse models [110] and is correlated with a poor prognosis in human HCC [123,124]. We identified both HLA-A24*(A*2402)* and H-2K^{d}-restricted GPC3$_{298\text{–}306}$ (EYIL-

SLEEL), as well as HLA-A2(*A*0201*)-restricted $GPC3_{144\text{-}152}$ (FVGEFFTDV), as peptides that can stimulate GPC3-reactive CTLs without inducing autoimmunity [110,125]. By performing a binding assay, we confirmed that the HLA-A*02:01-restricted $GPC3_{144\text{–}152}$ (FVGEFFTDV) peptide can also bind to HLA-A*02:06 and HLA-A*02:07. We also conducted a preclinical study in mice to design an optimal schedule for a clinical trial of the GPC3-derived peptide vaccine. This preclinical study showed that incomplete Freund's adjuvant (IFA) is indispensable for peptide-based immunotherapy, and that the immunological effect of the peptide vaccine was dose dependent [126].

4.2. Phase I clinical trial of a GPC3-derived peptide vaccine

Based on these results, we conducted a phase I clinical trial of this GPC3-derived peptide vaccine in patients with advanced HCC, the results of which were published recently [120]. Thirty-three advanced HCC patients were administered GPC3 vaccination intradermally (injections on days 1, 15, and 29 with dose escalation). $GPC3_{298\text{-}306}$ (EYILSLEEL) was used in HLA-A24-positive patients and $GPC3_{144\text{-}152}$ (FVGEFFTDV) in HLA-A2-positive patients. GPC3 peptide vaccination was well tolerated. One patient showed a partial response, and 19 showed stable disease 2 months after initiation of treatment. Four of the 19 patients with stable disease had tumor necrosis or regression that did not meet the criteria for a partial response. The disease control rate (partial response + stable disease) was 60.6%, 2 months after initiation of treatment. Levels of the tumor markers AFP and/or des-γ-carboxy prothrombin temporarily decreased in nine patients. We also analyzed the GPC3-specific CTL frequency by *ex vivo* IFN-γ enzyme-linked immunospot (ELISPOT) assay. In 30 patients, numbers of GPC3 peptide-specific CTLs increased in peripheral blood after GPC3 peptide vaccination. We established several $GPC3_{144\text{–}152}$ peptide-specific CTL clones with antigen-specific killing activity against tumor cells from PBMCs of patients vaccinated in this trial [119]. Tumor biopsies were performed (with informed consent) in seven patients to evaluate infiltration of CD8-positive T cells by immunohistochemical staining. Many CD8-positive T cells infiltrated tumors after vaccination. This study showed that the peptide-specific CTL frequency was correlated with overall survival in HCC patients receiving peptide vaccination. In multivariate analysis, the GPC3 peptide-specific CTL frequency was the predictive factor for overall survival in this trial. Analysis of all 33 patients showed that the median overall survival was 12.2 months (95% confidence interval, 6.5 to 18.0) in patients with high GPC3-specfic CTL frequencies, compared with 8.5 months (95% confidence interval, 3.7 to 13.1) in those with low GPC3-specfic CTL frequencies ($P = 0.033$). This study provided much immunological evidence that suggested the potential for improvement of overall survival.

4.3. Ongoing trials of GPC3-based immunotherapy

We subsequently conducted a phase II study of the GPC3-derived peptide vaccine as an adjuvant therapy for patients with HCC (University Hospital Medical Information Network Clinical Trials Registry, UMIN-CTR number: 000002614). Forty patients with initial HCC who had undergone surgery or radiofrequency ablation were enrolled in this phase II, open-label, single-arm trial. Ten vaccinations were performed over 1 year after curative treatment. The primary endpoints were the 1- and 2-year recurrence rates. The secondary endpoints were immunological responses, as measured by IFN-γ ELISPOT assay. Currently, the correlation between the time of recurrence and immunological responses is being analyzed.

We are conducting a subsequent trial for advanced HCC to assess whether TILs with an anti-tumor effect are indeed increased (UMIN-CTR number: 000005093). In all cases, liver biopsies will be performed before and after GPC3 peptide vaccination, according to the protocol. In the phase I trial, we did not confirm whether the TILs detected after vaccination were GPC3 peptide-specific. In the ongoing trial, we could detect GPC3 peptide-specific CTLs in liver biopsy specimens by flow cytometry using dextramer staining.

We expect that the results of these studies will validate the biomarkers and provide a rationale for a larger randomized clinical trial to determine the efficacy of the GPC3-derived peptide vaccine. Conversely, the antitumor effect in advanced cancer of the peptide vaccine alone is not dramatic. Thus, we aim to develop combinatorial approaches [127] or strong antigen-specific immunotherapies, such as ACT following lymphodepletion [20]. Additionally, clinical trials of the adoptive transfer of GPC3-specific CTLs in patients with HCC in Japan are planned [128].

5. Development of immunotherapy and potential of combined therapy

Combinatorial strategies could comprise either a combination of classic chemo- or radiotherapy or simultaneous application of different immunotherapeutic approaches. Many preclinical studies have shown synergistic effects of combined therapy, standard cytotoxic chemotherapy [127], or radiotherapy [129]. Elimination or inhibition of Treg activity by low-dose cyclophosphamide or antibodies against CD25 was shown to be a rational approach [130-132]. Simultaneous administration of antibodies against CTLA-4 [133] or PD-1[131] may modify the tumor immunosuppressive microenvironment, thereby increasing the efficacy of immunotherapy.

5.1. Potential of combination therapies

Some chemotherapeutic agents upregulate TAA expression or reduce tumor cell resistance to specific CTLs [134]. Subtoxic-dose chemotherapy increased the susceptibility of tumor cells to the cytotoxic effect of CTLs [127].

Cell-surface expression of MHC class I molecules was increased for many days in a radiation dose-dependent manner using a murine model [135]. Conversely, exposing HCC to low-dose radiation increases the efficacy of DC-mediated immunotherapy due to upregulation of MHC class II and Fas expression after irradiation [136].

HCC thermal ablation induced or enhanced T-cell responses specific for HCC–associated antigens in PBMCs derived from 20 patients with HCC [137]. Similarly, the effect on the immune system of radiofrequency ablation was greater than that of surgical resection in both HCC patients and tumor-bearing mice. All seven patients with GPC3-expressing HCCs exhibited an increase in GPC3-specific CTLs after radiofrequency ablation or TACE, but not after surgical resection [138].

5.2. Clinical trials of combinatorial approaches

Several clinical trials of combinational approaches have been reported.

Greten *et al*. reported the effect of low-dose cyclophosphamide treatment in combination with telomerase peptide (GV1001) vaccination in 40 patients with advanced HCC [139]. GV1001 treatment resulted in a decrease in the number of CD4+CD25+Foxp3+ Tregs; however, no GV1001-specific immune responses were detected after vaccination.

Conversely, a randomized phase II trial of a multiple tumor-associated peptide vaccine for renal cell carcinoma showed that a single dose of cyclophosphamide reduced the number of Tregs and that immune responders had prolonged survival if pretreated with cyclophosphamide (hazard ratio = 0.38; $P = 0.040$) [140]. There was no difference in survival of nonimmune responders in the cyclophosphamide and non-cyclophosphamide arms. Thus the synergistic effects of cyclophosphamide might require a specific immune response.

Nakamoto *et al*. reported that transcatheter arterial DC infusion into tumor tissues following transarterial embolization treatment was feasible and safe in 10 patients with cirrhosis and HCC [141]. There was a trend for patients infused with DCs to display a longer recurrence-free survival. Thus transcatheter arterial infusion might be rational for specifically inducing immune effects in the target lesion.

Thus far, few clinical trials of the combination of immunotherapy and chemotherapy in HCC have been reported because chemotherapy, with the exception of sorafenib therapy, has not been demonstrated to be useful. Further studies are necessary to increase the clinical efficacy of immunotherapy for advanced HCC. There is hope that the combination of well-designed clinical trials of innovative immunotherapeutic approaches will lead to development of efficient new therapies for treatment of HCC.

5.3. mAbs

Use of mAbs that target tumor antigens is an important therapeutic approach for cancer treatment. mAbs can act as both agonists and antagonists by binding important key receptors to control immune responses [142].

5.3.1. CD28

Antibodies against CD28 are known to induce antitumor immunity in combination with bi-specific antibodies that bind to both the tumor antigen and the TCR-CD3 complex [143]. However, CD28 antibodies can activate T cells directly, as shown in a phase I dose escalation trial using a CD28 mAb that reported severe toxicity, including a systemic inflammatory response. Thus infusion of CD28 mAbs is associated with serious difficulties [48].

5.3.2. CD137

CD137, a member of the TNF receptor superfamily, is expressed on antigen-activated T cells (CD4+,Cd8+ Tregs and NK cells), DCs, cytokine-activated NK cells, eosinophils, mast cells, and endothelial cells of some metastatic tumors, and binds to a high-affinity ligand expressed on several APCs such as macrophages and activated B cells [144]. An anti-CD137 mAb promoted survival of T cells and prevented cell death [145,146]. These suggest that anti-CD137 mAbs can enhance T cell-mediated immune responses. Melero *et al*. reported the antitumor effect of an anti-CD137 mAb on Ag104 sarcoma and P815 mastocytoma in mice [144].

Unfortunately, Niu *et al*. reported that single injection of anti-CD137 caused anomalies such as splenomegaly, hepatomegaly, lymphadenopathy, multifocal hepatitis, anaemia, altered trafficking of B cells and CD8+ T cells, loss of NK cells, and a 10-fold increase in bone marrow cells bearing the phenotype of hematopoietic stem cells [147].

5.3.3. OX40

OX40 (also known as CD134 and TNR4) is a member of the TNFR family that is expressed on activated CD4+ and CD8+ T cells. The OX40 ligand is expressed on activated APCs (DC, B cells, and macrophages), and possibly also on activated T cells and endothelial cells. OX40 ligand stimulates T-cell proliferation and ensures T-cell long-term survival. OX40 or OX40L deficiency leads to weaker CD4+ T-helper immune responses in mice. Moreover, expression of exogenous OX40L by tumor cells increases their immunogenicity, and causes their rejection by CD4+ T helper 1 cells and CTL responses. No side effects induced by OX40 ligand have yet been reported, although the possibility cannot be excluded because OX40 has been found on CD4+ lymphocytes infiltrating multiple sclerosis and inflammatory bowel disease lesions. Phase I clinical trials of a murine anti-human OX40 mAb have been initiated in patients with advanced cancer of multiple tissue origins, although repeat administration of this xenogeneic antibody will be limited due to immune responses against the murine sequences of the antibody [148].

5.3.4. GPC3

Chugai Pharmaceutical Co., Ltd. developed the GPC3 antibody (GC33) for treatment of HCC. They demonstrated antitumor efficacy of GC33 in several human liver cancer xenograft models and the important role of antibody-dependent cellular cytotoxicity (ADCC) in the antitumor mechanism of GC33. They also showed that macrophages play an important role in this antitumor activity, which is unlikely to be direct ADCC by macrophages themselves [149]. Clinical trials of GC33 in advanced HCC patients are ongoing.

5.3.5. CTLA-4

CTLA-4 is an immunosuppressive receptor on T cells. Via ligand binding, CTLA-4 generates inhibitory signals that reduce T-cell proliferation and IL-2 secretion. Administration of CTLA-4 mAbs demonstrated antitumor effects in some murine malignant models [150,151].

Prieto *et al*. followed patients with melanoma treated with CTLA-4 mAb (ipilimumab) and either the gp100 peptide or IL-2. Ipilimumab induced durable, potentially curative tumor regression in a small percentage of patients with metastatic melanoma; furthermore, combination with IL-2 increased the complete response rate [152]. Some phase II clinical trials have reported the safety and therapeutic effect of CTLA-4 mAb in HCC patients. CTLA-4 mAb showed promising antitumor effects against HCC in addition to antiviral activity against hepatitis C virus [153].

5.3.6. PD-1

PD-L1 is a member of the B7 family that can interact with programmed death-1 (PD-1). Its receptor PD-1 is expressed on activated T and B cells and elicits inhibitory signals [76]. A phase I trial using a fully human IgG4 PD-1 blocking antibody (MDX-1106) demonstrated objective responses with limited toxicity in patients with treatment-refractory solid tumors [154]. The objective responses of non-small cell lung cancer, melanoma, or renal-cell cancer associated with PD-1 antibody may be related to PD-L1 expression on tumor cells [77]. In HCC, PD-L1 expression is correlated with tumor aggressiveness and postoperative recurrence [155].

A number of other mAbs have demonstrated benefits for the treatment of HCC as well as undesired effects associated with their high affinity and selectivity. The most promising observations are that mAb therapies have synergistic effects in combination with other strategies.

6. Conclusion

To date, there is no report of adequate antitumor efficacy of immunotherapy in clinical trials involving advanced HCC patients. However, the available data suggest that immunotherapy has the potential to improve survival without impairing the quality of life, and is expected to be effective for prevention of recurrence.

Immunotherapy for HCC is still in the preclinical and clinical trial phases of development; however, it will become available and be clinically successful in the near future. Analysis of the correlation between clinical and immunological responses is required for to demonstrate the efficacy of immunotherapy. The challenge remains to design clinical trials to appropriately evaluate novel immunotherapies or combination therapies, and allow feedback to facilitate ongoing development.

Acknowledgements

This study was supported in part by Health and Labor Science Research Grants for Research on Hepatitis and for Clinical Research from the Ministry of Health, Labor, and Welfare, Japan.

Author details

Yu Sawada, Kazuya Ofuji, Mayuko Sakai and Tetsuya Nakatsura*

*Address all correspondence to: tnakatsu@east.ncc.go.jp

Division of Cancer Immunotherapy, Research Center for Innovative Oncology, National Cancer Center Hospital East, Kashiwa, Japan

References

[1] Llovet JM. Hepatocellular carcinoma.Lancet 2003; 362 1907-1917.

[2] Beaugrand M. Local/regional and systemic treatments of hepatocellular carcinoma. Semin Liver Dis 2005; 25 201-211.

[3] Bruix J. Management of hepatocellular carcinoma. Hepatology2005; 42 1208-1236.

[4] Llovet JM. Sorafenib in advanced hepatocellular carcinoma. N Engl J Med 2008; 359 378-390.

[5] Cheng AL. Efficacy and safety of sorafenib in patients in the Asia-Pacific region with advanced hepatocellular carcinoma: a phase III randomised, double-blind, placebo-controlled trial. Lancet Oncol 2009; 10 25-34.

[6] Morimoto M. Higher discontinuation and lower survival rates are likely in elderly Japanese patients with advanced hepatocellular carcinoma receiving sorafenib. Hepatol Res 2011; 41 296-302.

[7] Ryu M. Therapeutic results of resection, transcatheter arterial embolization and percutaneous transhepatic ethanol injection in 3225 patients with hepatocellular carcinoma: a retrospective multicenter study. Jpn J ClinOncol 1997; 27 251-257.

[8] Kumada T. Patterns of recurrence after initial treatment in patients with small hepatocellular carcinoma. Hepatology 1997; 25 87-92.

[9] Habu D. Role of vitamin K2 in the development of hepatocellular carcinoma in women with viral cirrhosis of the liver. JAMA 2004; 292 358-361.

[10] Muto Y. Prevention of second primary tumors by an acyclic retinoid, polyprenoic acid, in patients with hepatocellular carcinoma. Hepatoma Prevention Study Group. N Engl J Med 1996; 334 1561-1567.

[11] Ikeda K. Interferon beta prevents recurrence of hepatocellular carcinoma after complete resection or ablation of the primary tumor-A prospective randomized study of hepatitis C virus-related liver cancer. Hepatology 2000; 32 228-232.

[12] Kubo S. Effects of long-term postoperative interferon-alpha therapy on intrahepatic recurrence after resection of hepatitis C virus-related hepatocellular carcinoma. A randomized, controlled trial. Ann Intern Med 2001; 15(134) 963-967.

[13] Shiratori Y. Interferon therapy after tumor ablation improves prognosis in patients with hepatocellular carcinoma associated with hepatitis C virus. Ann Intern Med 2003; 138 299-306.

[14] ClinicalTrials.gov A service of the U.S. National Institute of Health. http://clinicaltrials.gov/ct2/show/NCT00692770 (accessed 30 August 2008).

[15] Breous E. Potential of immunotherapy for hepatocellular carcinoma. Journal of Hepatology 2011; 54 830–834.

[16] Greten TF. Immunotherapy of hepatocellular carcinoma. Journal of Hepatology 2006; 45 868–878.

[17] Takayama T. Adoptive immunotherapy to lower postsurgical recurrence rates of hepatocellular carcinoma: a randomised trial. Lancet 2000; 356 802-807.

[18] Kuang M. Phase II randomized trial of autologous formalin-fixed tumor vaccine for postsurgical recurrence of hepatocellular carcinoma. Clin Cancer Res 2004; 10 1574–1579.

[19] Peng BG. Tumor vaccine against recurrence of hepatocellular carcinoma. World J Gastroenterol 2005; 11 700–704.

[20] Rosenberg SA.Adoptive cell therapy for the treatment of patients with metastatic melanoma. CurrOpinImmunol. 2009;21(2) 233-240.

[21] Yoong KF. Phenotypic and functional analyses of fresh and recombinant interleukin-2 cultured tumour-infiltrating lymphocytes derived from malignant human liver tumours. BiochemSoc Trans. 1997;25(2) 271S.

[22] Wada Y.Clinicopathological study on hepatocellular carcinoma with lymphocytic infiltration.Hepatology 1998;27 407–414.

[23] Vollmer CM Jr. α -Fetoprotein-specifi c genetic immunotherapy for hepatocellular carcinoma. Cancer res 1999;59 (13) 3064 -3067

[24] Butterfield LH.T-cell responses to HLA-A*0201 immunodominant peptides derived from alpha-fetoprotein in patients with hepatocellular cancer. Clin Cancer Res. 2003;9(16 Pt 1) 5902-5908.

[25] Butterfield LH. A phase I/II trial testing immunization of hepatocellular carcinoma patients with dendritic cells pulsed with four α -fetoprotein peptides. Clin Cancer Res 2006;12(9) 2817-2825

[26] van der Bruggen P. A gene encoding an antigen recognized by cytolytic T lymphocytes on a human melanoma. Science1991; 254(5038) 1643–1647.

[27] Zerbini A. Ex vivo characterization of tumor-derived melanoma antigen encoding gene-specific CD8+ cells in patients with hepatocellular carcinoma. J Hepatol 2004; 40 (1) 102 -109

[28] Chen YT. Genomic cloning and localization of CTAG, a gene encoding an autoimmunogenic cancer-testis antigen NY-ESO-1, to human chromosome Xq28. Cytogenet.Cell Genet. 1997;79 237–240.

[29] Nakatsura T. Glypican-3, overexpressed specifically in human hepatocellular carcinoma, is a novel tumor marker. BiochemBiophys Res Commun 2003; 306 16-25.

[30] Villadangos JA. Intrinsic and cooperative antigen-presenting functions of dendritic-cell subsets in vivo. Nat Rev Immunol 2007;7 543–555.

[31] Carl G Figdor. Dendritic cell immunotherapy: mapping the way. Nature Medicine 2004;10(5) 475 - 480

[32] Bray SM. Dendritic cell-based vaccines positively impact natural killer and regulatory T cells in hepatocellular carcinoma patients. ClinDevImmunol. 2011;2011:249281.

[33] Belardelli F. Interferon-alpha in tumor immunity and immunotherapy. Cytokine Growth Factor Rev 2002;13 119-134.

[34] Singh RK. Interferons alpha and beta down-regulate the expression of basic fibroblast growth factor in human carcinomas. ProcNatlAcadSci U S A. 1995; 9;92(10) 4562-4566.

[35] Lin SM. Prospective randomized controlled study of interferon-alpha in preventing hepatocellular carcinoma recurrence after medical ablation therapy for primary tumors. Cancer 2004;100 (2) 376 -382.

[36] Sun HC. Postoperative interferon α treatment postponed recurrence and improved overall survival in patients after curative resection of HBV-related hepatocellular carcinoma: a randomized clinical trial. J Cancer Res ClinOncol 2006;132(7) 458-465.

[37] Patt YZ. Phase II trial of systemic continuous fluorouracil and subcutaneous recombinant interferon Alfa-2b for treatment of hepatocellular carcinoma. J ClinOncol 2003;21 421–427.

[38] Komorizono Y. Systemic combined chemotherapy with low dose of 5-fluorouracil, cisplatin, and interferon-alpha for advanced hepatocellular carcinoma: a pilot study. Dig Dis Sci 2003;48 877–881.

[39] Lygidakis NJ. Combined transarterial targeting locoregional immunotherapy–chemotherapy for patients with unresectable hepatocellular carcinoma: a new alternative for an old problem. J Interferon Cytokine Res 1995;15 467–72.

[40] Reinisch W. Prospective pilot study of recombinant granulocyte macrophage colony-stimulating factor and interferongamma in patients with inoperable hepatocellular carcinoma.J Immunother 2002;25 489–99.

[41] Gaffen SL. Overview of interleukin-2 function, production and clinical applications. Cytokine.2004;28(3) 109-23.

[42] Palmieri G. Ultra-low-dose interleukin-2 in unresectable hepatocellular carcinoma. Am J ClinOncol 2002;25 224-226.

[43] Aldeghi R. Low-dose interleukin-2 subcutaneous immunotherapy in association with the pineal hormone melatonin as a first-line therapy in locally advanced or metastatic hepatocellular carcinoma. Eur J Cancer 1994;30A 167-170.

[44] Köhler G. Continuous cultures of fused cells secreting antibody of predefined specificity. Nature. 1975;256(5517) 495-497.

[45] Galluzzi L. Trial Watch: Monoclonal antibodies in cancer therapy. Oncoimmunology. 2012;1(1) 28-37.

[46] Fife BT. Control of peripheral T-cell tolerance and autoimmunity via the CTLA-4 and PD-1 pathways. Immunol Rev 2008;224 166-182.

[47] Luhder F. Topological requirements and signaling properties of T cell-activating, anti-CD28 antibody superagonists. J Exp Med 2003;197 955-966.

[48] Suntharalingam G. Cytokine storm in a phase 1 trial of the anti-CD28 monoclonal antibody TGN1412. N Engl J Med. 2006;355(10) 1018-1028.

[49] Greenwald RJ.The B7 family revisited. Annu Rev Immunol 2005;23 515-48.

[50] Linsley PS. Human B7-1 (CD80) and B7-2 (CD86) bind with similar avidities but distinct kinetics to CD28 and CTLA-4 receptors. Immunity 1994;1 793-801.

[51] Pentcheva-Hoang T. B7-1 and B7-2 selectively recruit CTLA-4 and CD28 to the immunological synapse. Immunity 2004;21 401-413.

[52] Wolchok JD. Ipilimumabmonotherapy in patients with pretreated advanced melanoma:arandomised, double-blind, multicentre, phase 2, dose-ranging study. Lancet Oncol 2010;11 155-164.

[53] Hodi FS. Improved survival with ipilimumab in patients with metastatic melanoma. N Engl J Med 2010;363 711-723.

[54] Abe M, Thomson AW. Antigen processing and presentation in the liver. In: Gershwin ME, Vierling JM, Manns MP.(ed.)Liver Immunology Principles and Practice. Totowa: Humana Press Inc 2007;49-59.

[55] Knolle PA. Local control of the immune response in the liver.Immunol Rev 2000; 174 21–34.

[56] Crispe IN. Hepatic T cells and liver tolerance. Nat Rev Immunol 2003;3 51-62.

[57] Bissell DM,.Cell-specific expression of transforming growth factor-beta in rat liver.Evidence for autocrine regulation of hepatocyte proliferation. J Clin Invest 1995;96 447–455.

[58] De Minicis S. Gene expression profiles during hepatic stellate cell activation in culture and in vivo. Gastroenterology. 2007;132(5) 1937-1946.

[59] Gabrilovich D. Mechanisms and functional significance of tumour-induced dendritic-cell defects. Nat Rev Immunol 2004;4 941–952.

[60] Gabrilovich DI. Production of vascular endothelial growth factor by human tumors inhibits the functional maturation of dendritic cells. Nat Med. 1996;2(10) 1096-1103.

[61] Menetrier-Caux C. Inhibition of the differentiation of dendritic cells from CD34(+) progenitors by tumor cells: role of interleukin-6 and macrophage colony-stimulating factor. Blood 1998;92 4778–4791.

[62] Yang AS. Tumor-induced interleukin 10 suppresses the ability of splenic dendritic cells to stimulate CD4 and CD8 Tcell responses. Cancer Res 2003;63 2150–2157.

[63] Satthaporn S. Dendritic cells are dysfunctional in patients with operable breast cancer. Cancer ImmunolImmunother. 2004;53(6) 510-518.

[64] Ormandy LA. Direct ex vivo analysis of dendritic cells in patients with hepatocellular carcinoma. World J Gastroenterol 2006;12 3275–3282.

[65] Kurokohchi K. Expression of HLA class I molecules and the transporter associated with antigen processing in hepatocellular carcinoma. Hepatology 1996;23 1181-1188.

[66] Fujiwara K. Decreased expression of B7 costimulatory molecules and major histocompatibility complex class-I in human hepatocellular carcinoma. J GastroenterolHepatol 2004;19 1121-1127.

[67] Huang J. HLA class I expression in primary hepatocellular carcinoma. World J Gastroenterol. 2002;8(4) 654-657.

[68] Cheng J. Characterization of human Fas gene. Exon/intron organization and promoter region.J Immunol. 1995;154 1239–1245.

[69] Suda T. Molecular cloning and expression of the Fas ligand, a novel member of the tumor necrosis factor family.Cell. 1993;75 1169–1178.

[70] Curtin JF. Live and let die: regulatory mechanisms in Fas-mediated apoptosis. Cell Signal 2003,;15 983-992.

[71] Griffith TS. Fas ligand-induced apoptosis as a mechanism of immune privilege. Science 1995;270 1189-1192.

[72] Donald B. A role for CD95 ligand in preventing graft rejection. Nature 1995;377 630-632.

[73] Higaki K. Fas antigen expression and its relationship with apoptosis in human hepatocellular carcinoma and noncancerous tissues. Am J Pathol. 1996;149(2) 429-437.

[74] Jodo S. Elevated serum levels of soluble Fas/APO-1 (CD95) in patients with hepatocellular carcinoma. ClinExpImmunol 1998;112 166-171.

[75] Nagao M. The alteration of Fas receptor and ligand system in hepatocellular carcinomas: how do hepatoma cells escape from the host immune surveillance in vivo? Hepatology. 1999;30(2) 413-421.

[76] Agata Y. Expression of the PD-1 antigen on the surface of stimulated mouse T and B lymphocytes. IntImmunol. 1996;8765–8772.

[77] Topalian SL. Safety, activity, and immune correlates of anti-PD-1 antibody in cancer. N Engl J Med. 2012;366(26) 2443-2454.

[78] Shi F. PD-1 and PD-L1 upregulation promotes CD8(+) T-cell apoptosis and postoperative recurrence in hepatocellular carcinoma patients. Int J Cancer. 2011;128(4) 887-896.

[79] Wu K. Kupffer cell suppression of CD8+ T cells in human hepatocellular carcinoma is mediated by B7-H1/programmed death-1 interactions. Cancer Res 2009;69(20) 8067–8075.

[80] Chen C. Decoy receptor 3 overexpression and immunologic tolerance in hepatocellular carcinoma (HCC) development. Cancer Invest. 2008;26(10) 965-974.

[81] Shen HW. Overexpression of decoy receptor 3 in hepatocellular carcinoma and its association with resistance to Fas ligand-mediated apoptosis.World J Gastroenterol. 2005;11(38) 5926-5930.

[82] Ormandy LA. Increased populations of regulatory T cells in peripheral blood of patients with hepatocellular carcinoma.Cancer Res 2005;65 2457–2464.

[83] Yang XH. Increase of CD4(+)CD25(+) regulatory Tcells in the liver of patients with hepatocellular carcinoma. J Hepatol 2006;45(2) 254-262.

[84] Unitt E. Compromised lymphocytes infiltrate hepatocellular carcinoma: the role of T-regulatory cells. Hepatology 2005;41 722–730.

[85] Beckebaum S. Increased levels of interleukin-10 in serum from patients with hepatocellular carcinoma correlate with profound numerical deficiencies and immature phenotype of circulating dendritic cell subsets. Clin Cancer Res 2004;10 7260–7269.

[86] Lai CL. Recombinant interferon-alpha in inoperable hepatocellular carcinoma: a randomized controlled trial. Hepatology 1993;17 389-394.

[87] Ishikawa T. Immunotherapy of hepatocellular carcinoma with autologous lymphokine-activated killer cells and/or recombinant interleukin-2. J Cancer Res ClinOncol 1988;114 283-290.

[88] Qian C. Therapy of cancer by cytokines mediated by gene therapy approach. Cell Res 2006; 16 182-188.

[89] Trinchieri G. Interleukin-12 and the regulation of innate resistance and adaptive immunity. Nat Rev Immunol 2003; 3 133-146.

[90] Colombo MP. Interleukin-12 in anti-tumor immunity and immunotherapy. Cytokine Growth Factor Rev 2002; 13155-168.

[91] Sangro B. Gene therapy of cancer based on interleukin 12. Curr Gene Ther. 2005;5(6) 573-81.

[92] Lopez MV. IL-12 and IL-10 expression synergize to induce the immune-mediated eradication of established colon and mammary tumors and lung metastasis. J Immunol 2005; 175 5885-5894.

[93] Gilly FN. Gene therapy with Adv-IL-2 in unresectable digestive cancer: phase I-II study, intermediate report. Hepatogastroenterology 1999; 46(Suppl 1) 1268-1273.

[94] Garrido F. HLA class I antigens in human tumors. Adv Cancer Res 1995; 67 155–195.

[95] Schmidt W. Variation of expression of histocompatibility antigens on tumor cells:absence of H-2Kk-gene products from a gross virus-induced leukemia in BALB.K. Immunogenetics 1981; 14 323–339.

[96] Rubin J. Phase I study of immunotherapy of hepatic metastases of colorectal carcinoma by direct gene transfer of an allogeneic histocompatibility antigen, HLA-B7. Gene Ther 1997; 4 419-425.

[97] Liu TC. Gene therapy progress and prospects cancer: oncolytic viruses. Gene Ther 2008; 15(12) 877-884.

[98] Tani J. Update on current advances in gene therapy.West Indian Med J. 2011;60(2) 188-194.

[99] Bischoff JR. An adenovirus mutant that replicates selectively in p53-deficient human tumor cells. Science 1996; 274 373-376.

[100] Habib N. Clinical trial of E1B-deleted adenovirus (dl1520) gene therapy for hepatocellular carcinoma. Cancer Gene Ther 2002; 9 254-259.

[101] Sangro B. A phase 1 clinical trial of thymidine kinase-based gene therapy in advanced hepatocellular carcinoma. Cancer Gene Ther. 2010;17(12) 837-843.

[102] Kottke T. Antiangiogenic cancer therapy combined with oncolyticvirotherapy leads to regression of established tumors in mice. J Clin Invest. 2010; 120(5) 1551–1560.

[103] Zeyaullah M. Oncolytic Viruses in the Treatment of Cancer: A Review of Current Strategies. PatholOncol Res. 2012 Jun 20.

[104] Kawata A. Adjuvant chemoimmunotherapy for hepatocellular carcinoma patients. Adriamycin, interleukin-2, and lymphokine-activated killer cells versus adriamycin alone. Am J ClinOncol.1995;18(3) 257-62.

[105] TakayamaT . Distribution and therapeutic effect of intraarterially transferred tumor-infiltrating lymphocytes in hepatic malignancies. A preliminary report.Cancer. 1991;68(11) 2391-2396.

[106] Li Q. Adoptive T-cell immunotherapy of cancer.Cytokines Cell MolTher.1999;5(2) 105-17.

[107] Rosenberg SA. Adoptive cell transfer: a clinical path to effective cancer immunotherapy. Nat Rev Cancer 2008; 8 299-308.

[108] Grimm CF. Mouse alpha-fetoproteinspecific DNA-based immunotherapy of hepatocellular carcinoma leads to tumor regression in mice. Gastroenterology 2000; 119 1104-1112.

[109] Jeng YM. Overexpression and amplification of Aurora-A in hepatocellular carcinoma. Clin Cancer Res 2004; 10 2065-2071.

[110] Nakatsura T. Mouse homologue of a novel human oncofetal antigen, glypican-3, evokes T-cell-mediated tumor rejection without autoimmune reactions in mice. Clin Cancer Res 2004; 10 8630-8640.

[111] Liu FF.The specific immune response to tumor antigen CP1 and its correlation with improved survival in colon cancer patients.Gastroenterology 2008, 134 998-1006.

[112] Reis e Sousa C: Dendritic cells in a mature age. Nat Rev Immunol 2006; 6476-483.

[113] Chi KH.Combination of conformal radiotherapy and intratumoral injection of adoptive dendritic cell immunotherapy in refractory hepatoma. J Immunother 2005; 28 129-135.

[114] Iwashita Y. A phase I study of autologous dendritic cell-based immunotherapy for patients with unresectable primary liver cancer. Cancer ImmunolImmunother 2003; 52 155-161.

[115] Morse MA. A Phase I study of active immunotherapy with carcinoembryonic antigen peptide (CAP-1)-pulsed, autologous human cultured dendritic cells in patients with metastatic malignancies expressing carcinoembryonicantigen. Clin Cancer Res 1999, 5 1331-1338.

[116] Douglas J. gp100 Peptide Vaccine and Interleukin-2 in Patients with Advanced Melanoma.N Engl J Med 2011; 364 2119-2127.

[117] Perez SA. Results from a phase I clinical study of the novel Ii-Key/HER-2/neu(776-790) hybrid peptide vaccine in patients with prostate cancer. Clin Cancer Res. 2010 Jul 1;16(13) 3495-3506.

[118] ObaraW. Cancer Peptide Vaccine Therapy Developed from Oncoantigens Identified through Genome-wide Expression Profile Analysis for Bladder Cancer. Jpn J ClinOncol. 2012; 42(7) 591-600.

[119] Yoshikawa T. HLA-A2-restricted glypican-3 peptide-specific CTL clones induced by peptide vaccine show high avidity and antigen-specific killing activity against tumor cells.Cancer Sci. 2011; 102(5) 918-25.

[120] Sawada Y. Phase I Trial of a Glypican-3-Derived Peptide Vaccine for Advanced Hepatocellular Carcinoma: Immunologic Evidence and Potential for Improving Overall Survival. Clin Cancer Res. 2012; 18(13) 3686-3696.

[121] Mitchell H. Glypican-3: A new target for cancer immunotherapy. Euro J Cancer 2011; 47 333-338.

[122] Capurro MI. Glypican-3 promotes the growth of hepatocellular carcinoma by stimulating canonical Wnt signaling. Cancer Res 2005; 65 6245–6254.

[123] Shirakawa H. Glypican-3 is a useful diagnostic marker for a component of hepatocellular carcinoma in human liver cancer. Int J Oncol 2009; 34 649-656.

[124] Shirakawa H. Glypican-3 expression is correlated with poor prognosis in hepatocellular carcinoma. Cancer Sci 2009; 100 1403-1407.

[125] Komori H. Identification of HLA-A2- or HLA-A24-restricted CTL epitopes possibly useful for glypican-3-specific immunotherapy of hepatocellular carcinoma.Clin Cancer Res 2006; 12 2689-2697.

[126] Motomura Y. HLA-A2 and -A24-restricted glypican-3-derived peptide vaccine induce specific CTLs: preclinical study using mice. Int J Oncol 2008; 32 985-990.

[127] Suzuki S. Glypican-3 could be an effective target for immunotherapy combined with chemotherapy against ovarian clear cell carcinoma. Cancer Sci 2011; 102 1622-1629.

[128] Sawada Y.A glypican-3-derived peptide vaccine against hepatocellular carcinoma.OncoImmunology 2012; 1(8)1449-1551.

[129] Chakraborty M. Irradiation of tumor cells up-regulates Fas and enhances CTL lytic activity and CTL adoptive immunotherapy. J Immunol 2003; 170 6338-6347.

[130] Rico M. Low dose Cyclophosphmide (Cy) treatment induces a decrease in the percentage of regulatory T cells in lymphoma-bearing rats. Proc Am Assoc Cancer Res 2007; 48 233.

[131] Mkrtichyan M. Anti-PD-1 synergizes with cyclophosphamide to induce potent antitumor vaccine effects through novel mechanisms. Eur J. immunol 2011; 41 2977-2986.

[132] Liu Y. Adenovirus-mediated intratumoral expression of immunostimulatory proteins in combination with systemic Treg inactivation induces tumor-destructive immune responses in mouse models. Cancer Gene Ther. 2011; ;18(6)407-418.

[133] Peggs KS.Principles and use of anti-CTLA4 antibody in human cancer immunotherapy. Current Opinion in Immunology 2006; 18 206–213.

[134] Matar P. Immunotherapy for liver tumors: present status and future prospects Journal of Biomedical Science 2009, 16:30 doi:10.1186/1423-0127-16-30.

[135] Reits EA. Radiation modulates the peptide repertoire, enhances MHC class I expression, and induces successful antitumor immunotherapy. JEM 2006;203 1259-1271

[136] Lin CC. Potentiation of the immunotherapeutic effect of autologous dendritic cells by pretreating hepatocellular carcinoma with low-dose radiation.Clin Invest Med 2008; 31(3) 150-159.

[137] Zerbini A. Radiofrequency thermal ablation of hepatocellular carcinoma liver nodules can activate and enhance tumor-specific T-cell responses. Cancer Res 2006; 66 1139-1146.

[138] Nobuoka D. Radiofrequency ablation for hepatocellular carcinoma induces glypican-3 peptide-specific cytotoxic T lymphocytes. Int J Oncol 2012; 40 63-70.

[139] Greten TF. A phase II open trial evaluating safety and efficacy of a telomerase peptide vaccination in patients with advanced hepatocellular carcinoma. BMC cancer 2010; 10 209.

[140] Walter S. Multipeptide immune response to cancer vaccine IMA901 after single-dose cyclophosphamide associates with longer patient survival. Nat. Med. 2012 doi:10.1038/nm.2883

[141] Nakamoto Y. Combined therapy of transcatheter hepatic arterial embolization with intratumoral dendritic cell infusion for hepatocellular carcinoma: clinical safety. ClinExpImmunol 2007; 147 296-305.

[142] Zhu Y. Cancer therapeutic monoclonal antibodies targeting lymphocyte co-stimulatory pathways.CurrOpinInvestig Drugs 2003;4 691-695.

[143] Chen L. Costimulation of antitumor immunity by the B7 counterreceptor for the T lymphocyte molecules CD28 and CTLA-4. Cell 1992;71 1093-1102.,

[144] Melero I. Monoclonal antibodies against the 4-1BB T-cell activation molecule eradicate established tumors. Nat Med 1997;3 682-685.

[145] Shuford WW. 4-1BB costimulatory signals preferentially induce CD8+ T cell proliferation and lead to the amplification in vivo of cytotoxic T cell responses. J Exp Med 1997;186 47-55.

[146] Takahashi C. Cutting edge: 4-1BB is a bona fide CD8 T cell survival signal. J Immunol 1999;162 5037-5040.

[147] Niu L. Cytokine-mediated disruption of lymphocyte trafficking, hemopoiesis, and induction of lymphopenia, anemia, and thrombocytopenia in anti-CD137-treated mice. J Immunol 2007;178 4194-4213.

[148] Melero I. Immunostimulatory monoclonal antibodies for cancer therapy. Nat Rev Cancer 2007;7 95-106.

[149] Takai H. Histopathological analyses of the antitumor activity of anti-glypican-3 antibody (GC33) in human liver cancer xenograft models: The contribution of macrophages. Cancer BiolTher 2009; 10930-938.

[150] Leach DR. Enhancement of antitumor immunity by CTLA-4 blockade. Science 1996; 2711734-1736.

[151] Chambers CA. CTLA-4-mediated inhibition in regulation of T cell responses: mechanisms and manipulation in tumor immunotherapy. Annu Rev Immunol 2001; 19565-594.

[152] PrietoPA . CTLA-4 blockade with ipilimumab: long-term follow-up of 177 patients with metastatic melanoma. Clin Cancer Res. 2012;18(7) 2039-2047.

[153] Melero I. Antiviral and antitumoral effects of the anti-CTLA4 agent tremelimumab in oatients with hepatocellular carcinoma (HCC) and chronic hepatitis C virus infection: Results from a phase II clinical trial.:proceeding of the American Association for Cancer Research March 31- April 4 2012 McCormick Place West Chicago, IL

[154] Brahmer JR. Phase I study of single-agent anti–programmed death-1 (MDX-1106) in refractory solid tumors: safety, clinical activity, pharmacodynamics, and immunologic correlates. J ClinOncol 2010; 28: 3167-3175.

[155] Gao Q. Overexpression of PD-L1 significantly associates with tumor aggressiveness and postoperative recurrence in human hepatocellular carcinoma. Clin Cancer Res 2009; 15 971-979.

[156] Llovet JM.Randomized controlled trial of interferon treatment for advanced hepatocellular carcinoma.Hepatology 2000; 31:54-58.

[157] Ladhams A. Treatment of non-resectable hepatocellular carcinoma with autologous tumor-pulsed dendritic cells. J GastroenterolHepatol 2002; 17 889-896.

[158] Sakon M. Combined intraarterial 5-fluorouracil and subcutaneous interferon-alpha therapy for advanced hepatocellular carcinoma with tumor thrombi in the major portal branches. Cancer 2002; 94 435-442.

[159] Stift A. Dendritic cell-based vaccination in solid cancer. J ClinOncol 2003; 21 135-142.

[160] Feun LG. Recombinant leukocyte interferon, doxorubicin, and 5FUDR in patients with hepatocellular carcinoma-A phase II trial. J Cancer Res ClinOncol 2003; 129 17-20.

[161] Shi M. Autologous cytokine-induced killer cell therapy in clinical trial phase I is safe in patients with primary hepatocellular carcinoma. World J Gastroenterol 2004; 10 1146-1151.

[162] Sangro B. Phase I trial of intratumoral injection of an adenovirus encoding interleukin-12 for advanced digestive tumors. J ClinOncol 2004; 22 1389-1397.

[163] Lee WC. Vaccination of advanced hepatocellular carcinoma patients with tumor lysate-pulsed dendritic cells: a clinical trial. J Immunother 2005; 28 496-504.

[164] Kumagi T. Administration of dendritic cells in cancer nodules in hepatocellular carcinoma.Oncol Rep 2005; 14 969-973.

[165] Yin XY.Systemic chemo-immunotherapy for advanced-stage hepatocellular carcinoma.World J Gastroenterol 2005; 11 2526-2529.

[166] Mazzolini G. Intratumoral injection of dendritic cells engineered to secrete interleukin-12 by recombinant adenovirus in patients with metastatic gastrointestinal carcinomas. J ClinOncol 2005; 23 999-1010.

[167] Vitale FV. Hepatic intra-arterial interferon alpha 2b-based immunotherapy combined with 5-fluorouracil (5-FU)-based systemic chemotherapy for patients with hepatocellular carcinoma (HCC) not responsive and/or not eligible for conventional treatments: a pilot study. Anticancer Res 2007; 27 4077-4081.

[168] Weng DS. Minimally invasive treatment combined with cytokine-induced killer cells therapy lower the short-term recurrence rates of hepatocellular carcinomas. J Immunother 2008; 31 63-71.

[169] Hui D.A randomized, controlled trial of postoperative adjuvant cytokine-induced killer cells immunotherapy after radical resection of hepatocellular carcinoma.Dig Liver Dis 2009; 41 36-41.

[170] Palmer DH. A phase II study of adoptive immunotherapy using dendritic cells pulsed with tumor lysate in patients with hepatocellular carcinoma. Hepatology. 2009; 49(1) 124-132

[171] Olioso P. Immunotherapy with cytokine induced killer cells in solid and hematopoietic tumours: a pilot clinical trial. HematolOncol 2009; 27 130-139.

[172] Hao MZ. Efficacy of transcatheter arterial chemoembolization combined with cytokine-induced killer cell therapy on hepatocellular carcinoma: a comparative study. Chin J Cancer 2010; 29 172-177.

[173] Ma H. Therapeutic safety and effects of adjuvant autologous RetroNectin activated killer cell immunotherapy for patients with primary hepatocellular carcinoma after radiofrequency ablation.Cancer BiolTher. 2010; 9(11) 903-907.

[174] Zhou P. Phase I clinical study of combination therapy with microwave ablation and cellular immunotherapy in hepatocellular carcinoma. Cancer BiolTher. 2011; 11(5) 450-456.

Chapter 5

Primary Liver Tumours – Presentation, Diagnosis and Surgical Treatment

H. Bektas, H. Schrem, M. Kleine, A. Tamac,
F.W.R. Vondran, S. Uzunyayla and J. Klempnauer

Additional information is available at the end of the chapter

http://dx.doi.org/10.5772/55932

1. Introduction

Cystic lesions of the liver such as dysontogenic cysts and cystic disease of the liver, haemangioma, focal nodular hyperplasia (FNH), disturbed fat distribution of the liver, hamartoma and liver cell adenoma are summarized under the term primary benign hepatic tumours. On the other hand, malignant tumours of the liver are classified into primary and secondary tumours. Primary malignant hepatic tumours are hepatocellular carcinoma (HCC) and cholangiocellular carcinoma (CCC). In addition to the aforementioned tumours one also has to consider rare and very rare primary hepatic tumours, e.g. hemangioendothelioma and hepatosarcoma as well as hepatoblastoma in children. Secondary tumours of the liver, i.e. liver metastases, may result from various primary tumours located throughout the entire body and need to be discussed separately. Another important group of liver lesions are parasitic liver tumours, particularly Echinococcus cysticus and Echinococcus alveolaris, which also do not emanate primarily from the liver tissue.

From a surgeon's point of view, new scientific findings and developments in the surgical procedures of liver resection as well as additional emerging treatment strategies used for HCC, are worthy of note. Liver resection and liver transplantation as the surgical therapy options are competing with regard to the best clinical long-term results, but they complement each other in multimodal therapy concepts. Numerous new insights for the optimal concept of a multimodal therapy including surgical procedures, i.e. liver transplantation and liver resection, are to be expected. Life prolonging medical therapy with Sorafenib for advanced, inoperable HCC is particularly notable, highlighting an important medical therapy may play in the future development of multimodal treatment concepts. Laparoscopic procedures are used increasingly in liver surgery, and at least in the current literature, there is agreement that skills in laparoscopic surgery will not only be expected for cholecystectomy, but also increasingly for liver resection

2. Preoperative differential diagnosis of liver masses

2.1. Presentation and symptoms

An abdominal ultrasound scan (US) is used frequently as routine examination in patients presenting for a medical check-up or for clarification of symptoms such as upper abdominal pain, weight loss, anaemia, power loss, icterus and/or fever. However, these symptoms occur only in very advanced stages of malignant primary and secondary hepatic tumours.

Confirmed individual risk factors for HCC include age, alcohol abuse as well as concomitant or primary diseases, e.g. liver cirrhosis, non-alcoholic fatty degeneration of the liver (NASH), hemochromatosis, autoimmune hepatitis and chronic viral hepatitis B (HBV) or C (HCV). Interestingly, a case control study in a patient population from the M.D. Anderson Cancer Centers in Houston suggests that liver cirrhosis and chronic hepatitis C are also potential risk factors for the development of an intrahepatic CCC (Shaib YH et al.) This was not the case for extrahepatic CCC, although alcohol abuse per se, rather than cirrhosis or hepatitis, was reportedly a risk factor for both intra and extra hepatic CCC. Elevation of the tumour marker CA 19-9, as well as CA 50, was evident in approximately 60 % of cases with CCC.

Fever and chills are typical symptoms of bacterial cholangitis, which can occur with increasing frequency in primary sclerosing cholangitis (PSC). After a prolonged course, PSC is a known risk factor for both extrahepatic proximal bile duct carcinoma (Klatskin tumour, histologically CCC) and intrahepatic CCC. Frequently, icterus is the first symptom of a Klatskin tumour. In case of fever and evidence of a cystic liver mass, differentially a liver abscess has to be considered. If extrahepatic symptoms are present at the time of diagnosis of a liver cancer, such as deterioration of the general condition with weight loss, anaemia and/or weakness, one also has to consider a possible hepatic metastasis.

In females oral contraceptives are frequently discussed as a risk factor for the development of liver adenomas and FNH. Depending on the origin of the patient from an endemic area or after visits abroad, chronic hepatitis B or C as risk factors for liver cirrhosis as well as parasitic cystic liver diseases (e.g. echinococcosis) need to be considered. Intravenous drug abuse also is a known risk factor for chronic hepatitis B or C, which in turn are known risk factors for the development of liver cirrhosis and HCC.

2.2. Medical imaging and the role of preoperative fine-needle biopsy

In approximately 20 % of all routinely performed US of the abdomen liver masses are noted. Generally, these masses can be either benign, such as. cysts, hemangiomas, disturbed fat distribution, hamartomas, FNH and liver adenomas or malignant (See Table 1). Malignant masses include liver metastases and malignant primary liver tumours, e.g. HCC and CCC.

Particularly rare differential diagnoses are hepatoblastoma in children and in adults hepatic sarcoma and hemangioendothelioma.

After sonographic diagnosis of a liver mass other imaging procedures available for further differential diagnostic are US with contrast medium (CM), computer tomography (CT), magnetic resonance imaging (MRI), nuclear-medical procedures, US-guided liver biopsy and finally, the confirmation of the diagnosis following liver resection (Table 1).

Benign liver tumours	Characteristics demonstrated by radiological imaging
Cavernous haemangioma	Contrast medium-assisted US scan, CT, MRI: during the arterial phase discontinuous nodular enhancement at the tumour periphery followed by centripetal absorption of the contrast medium.
Liver cell adenoma	Under application of contrast medium early arterial wash-in and adaptation to the liver parenchyma in the late phase.
Focal nodular hyperplasia	Wheel spoke structure of the vascular architecture with central scar; under application of contrast medium star-shaped arterial vascularisation, homogenous adaptation to the liver parenchyma in the late phase.
Liver cysts	Conventional US: no echo, absence of a wall, dorsal intensified echo. In CT demonstration if septa and calcification in case of echinococcus.
Malignant liver tumours	**Characteristics demonstrated by radiological imaging**
Liver metastases	Good detection with US scan, CT and MRI. Very variable presentation.
Hepatocellular carcinoma	Early arterial hypervascularisation with quick wash-out during the parenchymal phase.
Cholangiocellular carcinoma	Difficult to detect, use of multimodal radiological imaging methods makes sense (US, CT, MRI, when suspecting a Klatskin tumour ERCP).

Table 1. Characteristics of focal liver masses in radiological imaging.

Today, presentation combined with medical imaging enables us to obtain the correct diagnosis in more than 90 % of cases before the final histological result is available. The algorithm depicted in Figure 1 shows the diagnostic approach under inclusion of modern imaging procedures.

Basically it would be most preferable to have an almost positive differential diagnosis prior to commencing surgery, particularly as extensive liver resection involves considerable risks, which are to be taken seriously. Furthermore, the choice of the best possible multimodal therapy often depends on the differential diagnosis of the malignant tumours. To date, incorporation of the surgical treatment options liver resection and liver transplantation in an interdisciplinary treatment concept can be considered as a standard. As presented below, this interdisciplinary treatment concept can vary considerably depending on the type of liver tumour diagnosed and possible additional diseases of the parenchyma, e.g. liver cirrhosis.

As a specialized centre for liver resection and transplantation, we personally have found cases in which, contrary to the results of the preoperative imaging, diagnosis of a malignant tumour could not be confirmed in the final histology. It is not rare that instead of the suspected HCC

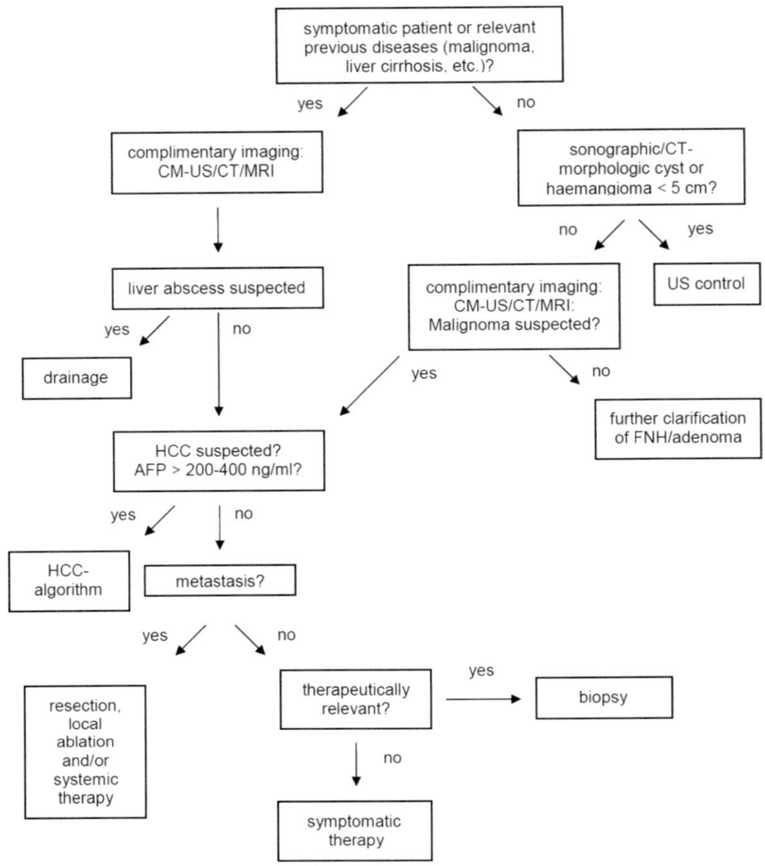

Figure 1. Algorithm for the clarification of a focal liver lesion (For HCC-algoritm see Fig 4 or EORTC EASL 2012)

the final histology shows an adenoma or intrahepatic haematoma, a haemangioma or a comparatively harmless hamartoma, none of which require urgent surgical treatment. The quality of the current preoperative radiological diagnostic together with the determination of the tumour marker alpha-fetoprotein (AFP) and the patient's anamnesis does not necessarily require a preoperative histological confirmation with fine-needle biopsy of the diagnosis of malignant liver tumour. Due to possible false negative results and the risk of potential implantation metastases in the puncture channel, today frequently a fine-needle biopsy is explicitly not desired. Therefore, one has to expect cases in which the preoperatively assumed malignancy is not confirmed histologically in the resection sample. In view of this fact, patients should be informed explicitly of this small but still existing risk. However, it has to be pointed out that in patients with a new liver mass and a history of a malignant tumour, the probability is great that this mass is a metastasis. In patients with the typical risk constellations for HCC, e.g. liver cirrhosis or chronic HBV or HCV or hemochromatosis, the risk of the new liver mass being a HCC is considerably higher, even when the serum AFP value is not verifiably elevated. In cases of doubt, an US-guided fine-needle biopsy makes sense, although it has to be considered that a negative histology cannot positively exclude a malignant tumour.

3. Indication for surgery for primary liver tumours

Primary malignant liver tumours and liver metastases are the most frequent indications for liver resection. When liver resection is indicated the patient's general condition and the comorbidity must not be disregarded. Particularly patients with cardiovascular and pulmonary diseases should receive the appropriate optimal treatment for these conditions prior to the planned liver resection to minimize the general risks, especially the post-surgical mortality. Preoperatively, it should be made absolutely clear to the patient that it is vital to avoid exposure to hepatotoxic substances, e.g. alcohol, paracetamol and drugs and preferably also to refrain from smoking. When deciding on the indication disease-specific aspects are also to be considered, e.g. type of liver tumour and degree of possible concomitant diseases of the liver parenchyma (Figure 1).

3.1. Evaluation of the risk of postoperative liver failure after liver resection and clarification of a possible indication for liver transplantation

Prior to any liver resection it is vital that the liver function is checked. If impaired liver function is evident (e.g. reduced serum cholinesterase or prothrombin time (PT), or elevated INR value without causal anticoagulative medication), an additional liver parenchyma disease should either be diagnosed or excluded (e.g. fatty liver, viral hepatitis, liver cirrhosis, NASH, hemochromatosis etc.). As a rule, these conditions have a considerable influence on the risk for potentially lethal postoperative liver failure. Further morphological indirect signs of a possible additional disease of the parenchyma are ascites and evidence of circulatory collaterals; these can be seen in either Doppler-US or CT of the abdomen.

Preoperatively unknown thrombocytopenia or hyperbilirubinaemia should also give cause to consider an additional liver disease other than a liver tumour. In such cases it is urgently recommended to consult an experienced hepatologist for detailed diagnostic purposes. Should in addition to the HCC a parenchymal disease and impaired liver function be diagnosed, depending on the individual case, the surgical treatment option should be liver transplantation instead of resection. In any case, such patients should be referred to a liver centre that can offer all relevant therapy modalities, including transplantation, for the treatment of HCC. Disregard of these basic principles can result in fatal errors, which can lead to the surgeon being confronted with a potentially preventable and difficult to treat postoperative liver failure. In addition, the surgeon would be unaware of the exact parenchymal damage that was the essential contributor; neither would he be in a position to consider liver transplantation as a possible alternative.

Today, the generally accepted standard in most cases is interdisciplinary treatment and a multimodal therapy concept. When combining multimodal therapy concepts with liver resection, the general rule is to adhere to an interval of at least 4-6 weeks between chemotherapy and planned liver resection. This is vital to minimize the risk of postoperative liver failure as sequelae of resection combined with a more or less hepatotoxic chemotherapy. Such an interval will allow time for physiological liver regeneration instead of unnecessarily endangering regeneration through possibly still active cytostatic effects of the chemotherapy.

If extended liver resection is indicated and a remaining liver volume is expected to be small, means of minimizing the risk of postoperative liver failure should be considered, e.g. hypertrophy of the remaining liver tissue. When considering that this may be necessary, it can be useful in individual cases to perform volumetry with using digital CT-, MRI- or US-data to determine the remaining liver volume in relation to the liver volume to be resected.

Particularly difficult is the preoperative assessment and prediction of the function of the liver tissue remaining after resection, especially when extended resection is necessary, with the possibility of additional damage to the liver parenchyma. It is catastrophic for the patient and his relatives, as well as for the liver surgeon, if after liver resection the remaining liver 'fails' as a result of the so-called small-for-size syndrome. This syndrome has a high mortality. Currently, it is still impossible to forecast accurately the probable function of the remaining liver tissue. Here the surgeon's skills and experience still play a prominent role. Particularly in patients with malignant tumours for whom the primary liver transplantation as alternative to liver resection is out of the question (e.g. CCC or non-neuroendocrine liver metastases), the possible risk of a potentially lethal failure of the remaining liver tissue after surgery has to be discussed in detail with the patients and their relatives. In principle, when informing the patients of risks and chances of liver resection, this problem should also be discussed in detail. In some cases of postoperative liver failure after resection an emergency liver transplantation save life, if a suitable organ becomes available in time. Of course, it cannot be assumed that this presents a realistic option in each case of failure of the remaining liver tissue.

Fortunately, it is rarely the case that the established radiological and laboratory-chemical methods do not show any signs of a cirrhotic liver and cirrhosis is primarily discovered during surgery. If the standard preoperative preparations were performed, it is our opinion that it is not necessarily a treatment error if the diagnosis of liver cirrhosis is initially made during surgery. The reason for this being that it is widely known that in many cases there are only indirect clinical signs. Generally, cirrhosis only becomes clinically notable at the advanced stage, and ultimately can only be confirmed histologically as currently routine preoperative liver biopsy cannot be generally recommended.

3.2. Neuroendocrine liver tumours

In the case of liver metastases of neuroendocrine tumours, e.g. those rare primary neuroendocrine liver tumours, which however are usually metastases of a still undiagnosed primary tumour, instead of liver resection there is the alternative of liver transplantation. However, it has to be noted that according to the presently valid and binding guidelines of the Federal Medical Council liver transplantation is permitted as an option for neuroendocrine liver metastases after potentially curatively resected primary tumour. These guidelines categorically rule out liver transplantation as a treatment option for other liver metastases, e.g. for the comparatively frequent colorectal liver metastases.

3.3. Intrahepatic cholangiocellular carcinoma and Klatskin tumour

As currently there are no other potential curative therapy options for CCC (Figure 2), e.g. radiation treatment or chemotherapy, one should consider the indication for liver resection rather liberally. This also applies for the intrahepatic CCC and the proximal bile duct carcinoma at the hepatic bifurcation, the so-called Klatskin tumour. Particularly in the case of a Klatskin tumour it is necessary to take the risk to perform only an exploratory laparotomy. Especially this tumour frequently permits only intraoperatively to determine definitively whether it is technically viable with a justifiable risk and whether resection is potentially curative. In some cases one can only determine after the resection of the hepatic bifurcation and affected liver lobe that ultimately histologically tumour-free resection margins are not feasible without risking failure of the residual liver by a too greatly extended liver resection. In this context one has to consider that depending on the extent of resection, connecting the intrahepatic bile ducts of the 3rd order or bile ducts located even further peripheral to a biliodigestive anastomosis becomes increasingly more difficult or technically surgical impossible. The intraoperative assessment of the extent of resection necessary must in these cases clearly be left to the experience of the operating surgeon. In our opinion it is certainly not a treatment error to complete the intervention as R1-resection. We consider that in the case of a Klatskin tumour it is rather the question whether or not refusal of referral to a centre particularly experienced in the field of hepatobiliary surgery for an explorative laparotomy is regarded as a possible treatment error, e.g. in the sense this may be considered as refusing any patient his legitimate right to an indicated operation. It should always be kept in mind that for a Klatskin tumour there are no other surgical options with a potential perspective for long-term survival, and it is our experience that as a rule it is impossible to recognize whether or not a curative resectability of a Klatskin tumour is feasible solely by means of radiological imaging. It can occur that a patient with PSC develops a proximal bile duct carcinoma, e.g. a Klatskin tumour, while waiting for liver transplantation, or is suspected as the result of the cytological examination of epithelial tissue of the bile duct. Today, these patients still have the option of liver transplantation as well as the option of an application to EUROTRANSPLANT for an upgrade of the urgency based on the match MELD score. This could probably shorten the time on the waiting list for a donor organ. In such cases neglecting to submit to EUROTRANSPLANT the application for an upgrade of the match MELD score could possibly be considered as a treatment error. However, this option is currently not available to patients with a Klatskin tumour due to poor experience regarding their long-term course.

In case of an intrahepatic CCC it is unquestionable that liver resection is the only potential curative method of treatment and thus should always be intended despite the generally high risk associated with the surgical intervention, e.g. due to a congruently marked comorbidity. According to the currently valid and binding guidelines of the Federal Medical Council liver transplantation is no longer a treatment option available to patients with intrahepatic CCC; this decision is based on the poor experiences made in the past regarding the long-term courses of these patients.

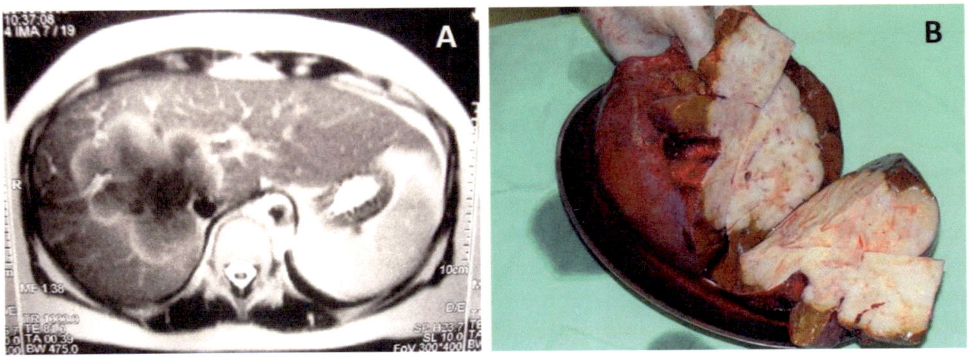

Figure 2. MRI scan (**A**) and surgical specimen (**B**) of a cholangiocellular carcinoma (CCC).

3.4. Hepatocellular Carcinoma (HCC)

For the treatment of HCC (Figure 3) the indication for resection and liver transplantation should be highly differentiated. One also has to consider alternative or complimentary therapeutic methods, which should or could be adopted multimodal with resection or transplantation (Figure 4). Here are meant particularly transarterial chemoembolisation (TACE), radio-frequency induced thermoablation (RITA) and percutaneous ethanol instillation (PEI) as well as chemotherapy with the protein kinase inhibitor Sorafenib.

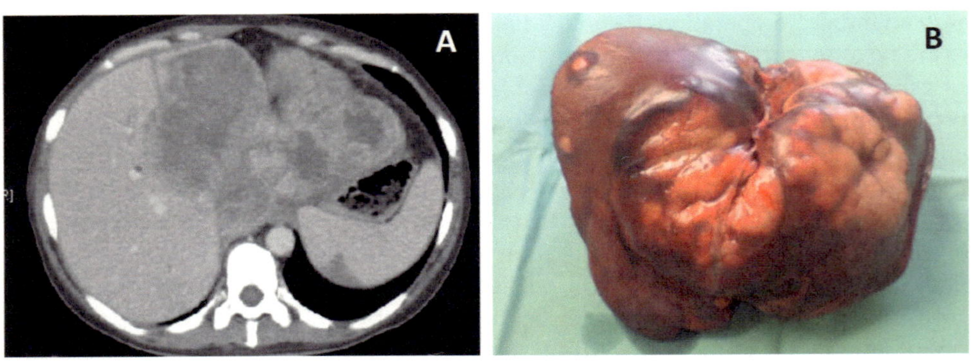

Figure 3. CT scan (**A**) and surgical specimen (**B**) of a hepatocellular carcinoma (HCC) without liver cirrhosis.

The interventional methods, e.g. TACE, RITA and PEI should be used in close interdisciplinary context with the surgical treatment options and be applied according to the individual case (Figure 4). Further consideration has to be given to additional diseases of the liver parenchyma, e.g. fatty liver, liver fibrosis, cirrhosis and hepatitis (viral hepatitis B and C, autoimmune hepatitis, NASH). Not to be disregarded is the drug treatment already applied for these conditions as this may have an influence on the risk of liver failure after liver resection or other interventions and in the case of a HCC this could well be an indication

http://dx.doi.org/10.5772/55932

for liver transplantation. Furthermore, a prerequisite should be the most exact tumour staging possible with the modern imaging methods, e.g. to enable a positive exclusion of extrahepatic tumour growth or vascular infiltration prior to reaching the indication. Close interdisciplinary cooperation in the liver transplantation centre with regularly held case discussions has proven to be essential regarding avoidance of erroneous indications. Today such close interdisciplinary cooperations, including regular case discussions, should be made a requirement for the treatment of HCC.

For patients with HCC, liver transplantation presents a potentially curative therapy option depending on the tumour stage at the time of transplantation. However, in most transplantation centres the precondition is that these patients have to fulfil the so-called Milan criteria to be accepted on the waiting list (no extrahepatic tumour growth, exclusion of infiltration of the portal vein, a maximum of 3 tumour nodules with diameter of less than 3 cm, the size of a single tumour nodule must be less than 5 cm).

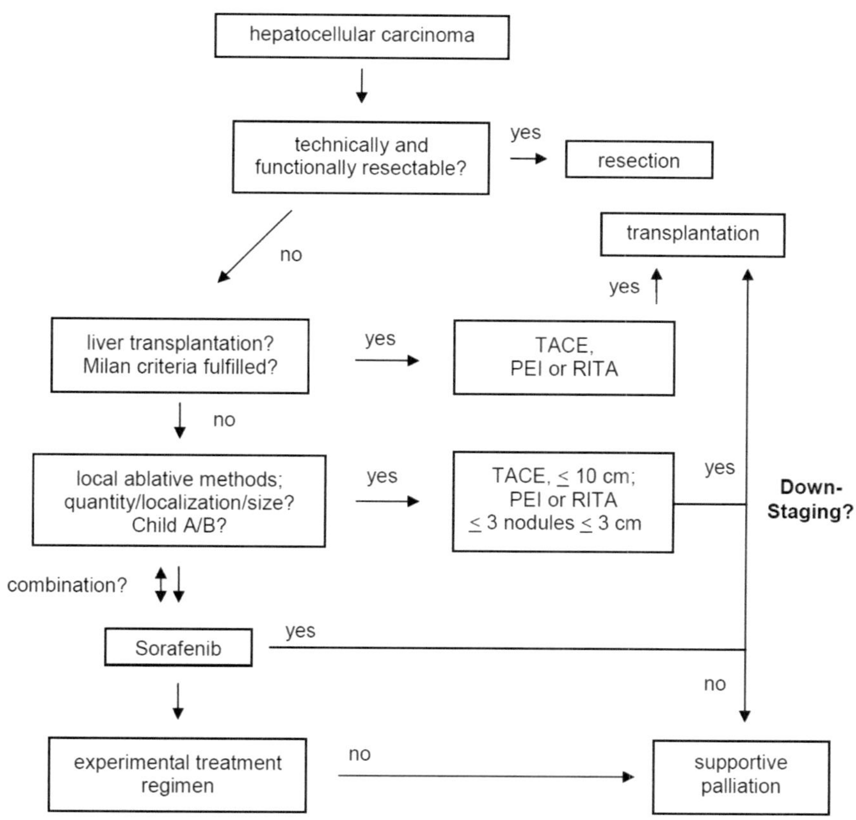

Figure 4. Algorithm for the therapy of hepatocellular carcinoma (HCC).

Liver transplantation is the treatment of first choice for selective patients with HCC, e.g. patients who are not candidates for resection and with tumour growth limited to the liver only. With transplantation optimal results can be achieved in patients with single lesions (diameter 2 – 5 cm or no more than 3 lesions with a max. diameter of 3 cm) without radiolocal evidence of extrahepatic tumour spread (Figures 5a/b). To achieve optimal results in patients with the above mentioned characteristics, it is imperative that a donor organ becomes available within 6 months (Figures 5c).

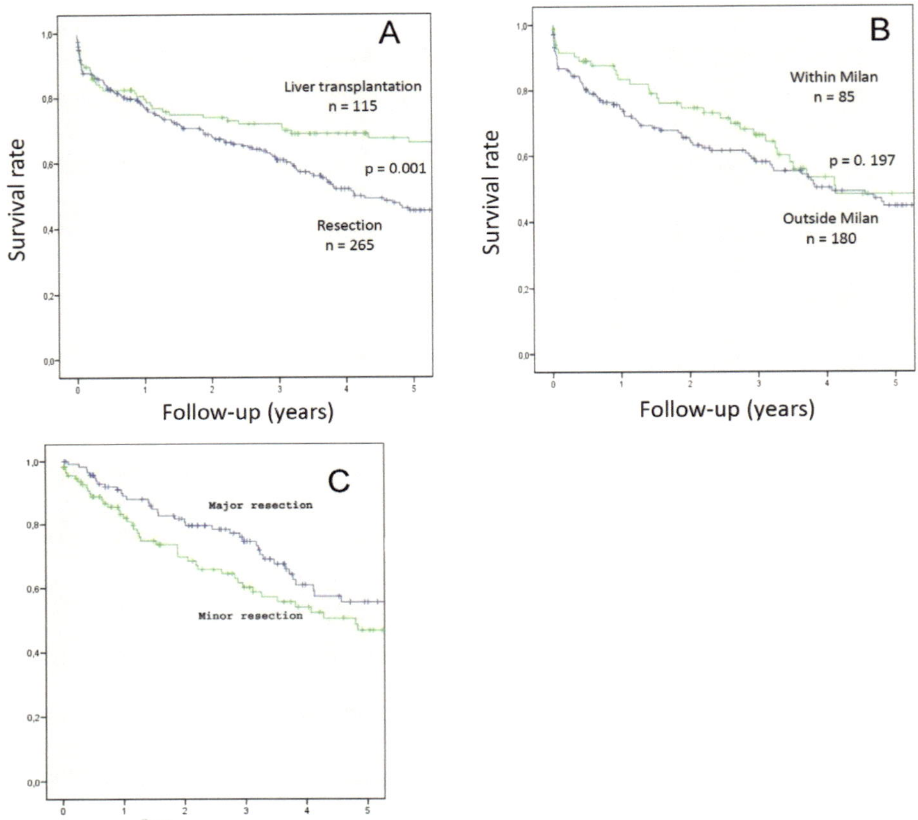

Figure 5. Outcome of surgical treatment for HCC: liver resection vs. liver transplantation (**A**), liver resection within Milan criteria vs. outside Milan criteria (**B**) and liver resection vs. explorative laparotomy only (**C**), for the years 1995 to 2006 at the Hannover Medical School.

The evident lack of donor organs from brain-dead donors regularly raises the question regarding the significance of liver donation from a living donor for patients with HCC. This discussion becomes particularly difficult when a healthy and suitable relative volunteers to donate part of his/her liver for a patient with HCC and an unfavourable prognosis (patient does no longer fulfil the characteristics necessary for a good prognosis after liver transplantation due to advanced tumour spread). In such situations the surgical risk for the healthy donor obviously becomes distinctly more important, and it is our opinion that in most of these cases transplantation is no longer ethically justifiable. Additionally, it has to be considered that a considerably longer waiting period for a matching donor organ (>1 year) has to be expected. Obviously, a great problem is the tumour progress while the patient waits for liver transplantation. TACE of HCC nodules is an established treatment method to prevent tumour progress and is used also frequently in our centre. A meta-analysis of all cohort trials and all prospective trials regarding TACE alone or in combination with additional percutaneous ablative interventions published in PubMed was recently performed. The result of this analysis was TACE alone performed in HCC patients prior to liver transplantation can effectively reduce the number of patients lost (so-called drop-outs) due to tumour progress while on the waiting list as they no longer fulfil the criteria for transplantation. The analysis also showed that a combined application of TACE and other percutaneous ablative methods can improve survival. It appears that a multimodal approach may provide the best results in the treatment of HCC.

For the surgical therapy of HCC the safety margin to be chosen for the resection plays a significant role for the surgeon. A prospective, randomised study performed in China compared a small (1 cm) with a large (2 cm) safety margin in a total of 169 patients in the sense of an intention-to-treat approach. The study showed that aiming for a safety margin of 2 cm lead to significantly improved survival rates after 1, 2, 3 and 5 years (Shi et al).

The results of the second interim analysis of the randomised Sorafenib study were published in the New England Journal of Medicine in 2008 (Llovet et al.) As the treatment with Sorafenib already showed significant advantages regarding the survival of patients with advanced HCC and the time span until progress was radiologically evident, the study was discontinued after the second interim analysis. Considering multimodal therapy concepts, these results will probably be relevant for the surgical treatment of HCC in the future. Currently, there are no study results that can show which role Sorafenib can play in adjuvant or neoadjuvant therapy concepts. A meta-analysis could show that patients treated with an adjuvant interferon therapy after liver resection due to HCC with concomitant viral hepatitis had a significant advantage regarding survival and tumour recurrence. This result is also supported by another meta-analysis concerning the same question. A retrospective analysis performed in France investigated the results after liver resection in patients with HCC, who fulfilled the Milan criteria at the time of resection. Here it could be shown that in case of recurrence after resection 61% of patients could be transplanted successfully (intention-to-treat analysis) (Bhangui et al., 2011).

3.5. Liver adenoma

For the principally benign liver adenoma (Figure 6) resection is generally indicated, when the adenoma measures >4 cm in diameter. The main reason for this is that an increase in diameter will raise the danger of a rupture. Furthermore, there is a risk of malignant degeneration in adenomas, although this can be hard to assess. Small adenomas can be mistaken for carcinomas, while needle biopsies suggesting and adenoma can be falsely negative.' Ultimately, the fine-needle biopsy only presents a random sample, which cannot exclude safely a malignant tumour if there is no evidence in the biopsy material.

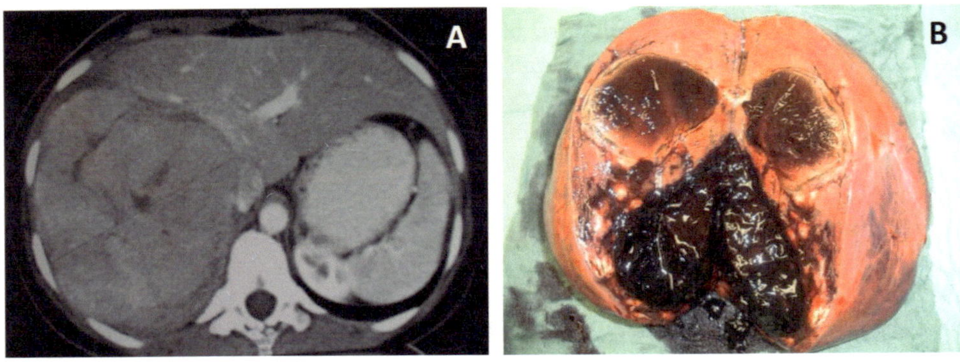

Figure 6. CT scan (**A**) and surgical specimen (**B**) of a partially hemorrhagic liver adenoma.

An American investigation analyzed retrospectively data of 5 hepatobiliary centres. A total of 124 mainly female patients were included, who were treated for liver adenomas between 1997 and 2006. The study resulted in the recommendation that patients with asymptomatic liver adenomas, which are >4 cm and/or patients taking contraceptive drugs therapy should undergo resection (Deneve et al.). A histopathological study performed in Bordeaux showed that the activation of beta-catenin in liver cell adenomas is associated with an increased risk to develop a HCC (Bioulac-Sage et al.)

3.6. *Dysontogenic cysts, Echincoccus cysticus* and *Echinococcus alveolaris*

Cystic liver tumours are either dysontogenetic cysts, biliary adenomas or infectious liver cysts. In principle, a cystic liver disease has to be considered differential diagnostically. Dysontogenetic liver cysts (solitary or multiple cysts) are benign, and approximately 1-7% of the ordinary population are affected. Most of these cysts are harmless and will only become symptomatic with increasing size. One has to differentiate between these normally solitary cysts and cystic liver disease. In cystic liver disease the complete liver is virtually infiltrated by cysts. During the late stage, when the patient becomes cachetic and liver failure is imminent, the therapy is liver transplantation. In most cases liver cysts are found incidentally when performing an abdominal US. Morphologically, the cysts show a smooth outline with a clear, liquid content (Figure 7). The walls of these cysts are delicate without calcification. The symptoms are mostly pain in the liver capsule with a sensation of pressure in the upper abdomen. However, considerable vascular compression can occur, e.g. compression of the retrohepatic caval vein or the portal vein. Frequently symptoms also result in compression of the stomach causing stenosis of cardia or pylorus as well as a displacement of neighbouring organs.

When echinococcosis is suspected, a serological exclusion or confirmation is required. Surgical therapy is indicated only when an increasing size causes symptoms or infections occur recurrently. Apart from open or laparoscopic marsupialisation or pericystectomy, partial resection of the liver is also a surgical treatment option. In most cases a simple liberal marsupialisation of the cyst is completely adequate to eliminate the symptoms permanently.

http://dx.doi.org/10.5772/55932

However, it is important to ensure that the marsupialisation is performed in such a way that secondary adhesion of the roof of the cyst with subsequent persisting or recurring symptoms do not occur. Naturally, pericystectomy is not associated with this danger, but with a higher risk for a secondary haemorrhage or development of a bile leakage and therefore should only be performed in exceptional cases.

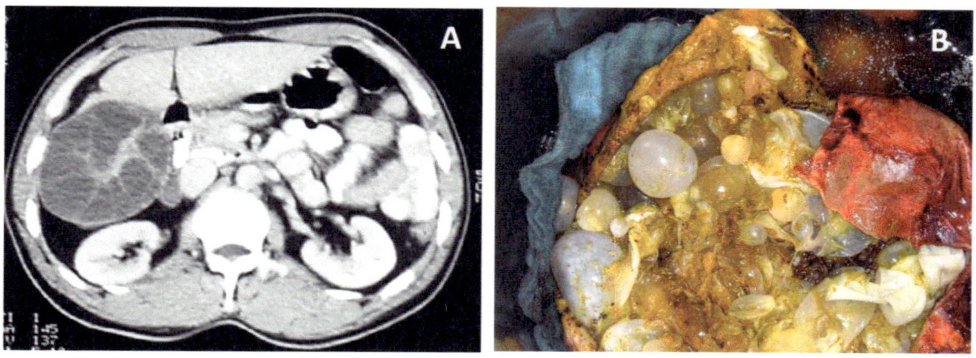

Figure 7. CT scan (**A**) and surgical specimen (**B**) of an Echinococcus granulosus cyst within the liver.

For the surgical treatment of Echinococcus cysticus a pericystectomy can be considered state-of-the-art. Echinococcus alveolaris requires an anatomical liver resection with an adequate safety margin similar to when resecting a malignant tumour. State-of-art surgical treatment for a large dysontogenetic liver cyst is marsupialisation. To perform a marsupialisation for cystic echinococcosis is obviously not per se treatment error, but due to the high risk of recurrence it is no longer performed by us and remains only an option in special cases. With respect to the surgical method applied treatment errors can occur when an Echinococcus cysticus is mistaken for an Echinococcus alveolaris or a harmless large liver cyst. Another reason for the wrong surgical procedure chosen may result when a preoperative echinococcus serology was not performed. This can result in marsupialisation of what is assumed to be a simple liver cyst with dissemination of still viable larvae into the free abdominal cavity, and often the catastrophic sequelae is a disease in the peritoneal cavity due to their free dissemination. Furthermore, the cysts can be joined to bile ducts. Therefore, when treating echinoccus cysts one should refrain from injecting high proof ethanol or formalin to destroy live larvae. Due to bile duct toxicity of ethanol or formalin these substances could cause secondary sclerosing cholangitis with subsequent chronic liver failure necessitating liver transplantation. In view of this risk, we necessarily consider injecting echinococcus cysts with high proof ethanol or formalin using the so-called PAIR method (Puncture – Aspiration – Injection – Reaspiration) as problematic, whereas the injection of 10% NaCl solution or 40% glucose solution by the so-called PAIR method to kill any viable larvae appears more justifiable.

3.7. Primary malignant hepatic hemangioendothelioma (hypertrophic endothelioma)

The etiology of these rare vascular tumours is unknown and the clinical appearance extremely variable. Data published show that in most patients a diffuse bilobate affected liver was evident, and thus the treatment was liver transplantation (44.8%). Whereas 24.8 % of patients received no treatment, 21 % received chemotherapy or radiation treatment and 9.4 % of patients underwent liver resection (Meharabi et al.). After liver transplantation the mean 1-year survival rate was 96 % and the mean 2-year survival rate was 54.5 %. Whereas the 1-year survival rate of untreated patients was 39.3 % and the 5-year survival rate was 4.5 %. After 1 year the survival rate of patients treated with chemotherapy and radiation was 73.3 % and 30% after 5 years, whereas the 1-year survival rate of patients who underwent resection was 100 % and the 5-year survival rate of still 75 %. Therefore, liver resection has to be the first choice for patients with resectable tumours, liver transplantation should be the first choice if both liver lobes are diffusely affected and there are no extrahepatic metastases.

3.8. Cavernous haemangioma

The cavernous haemangioma is the most frequently occurring benign hepatic tumour (absolute frequency of 0.5-7 % among the normal population), with a slight predominance in females (Galanski et al). The majority of these tumours are found accidentally by US scan. In most cases they cause no clinical symptoms, but become symptomatic once they increase in size. The symptoms caused by compression and displacement of blood vessels and neighbouring organ are similar to those experienced by dysontogenic liver cysts. Apart from US, other diagnostic methods used are MRI and CT (Figure 8). If further clarification is required, blood pool scintiscanning can be used as an additionally diagnostic tool. The only indication for surgical intervention is when the cavernous haemangioma becomes symptomatic. Generally, the danger of a haemorrhage caused by an accident, e.g. blunt abdominal trauma with ruptur of the cavernous haemangioma, is considered negligible, but cannot be categorically excluded. Ideally, whenever possible a haemangioma should be enucleated, e.g. this can be conducted in total vascular occlusion. When enucleation is impossible, the surgical treatment has to be resection of the appropriate section of the liver. It is vital to bear in mind the possibility of bile ducts being inside the wall of the haemangioma. Consequently, there is a significant risk ofbile leakage during enucleation.

During the last 10 years 49 patients (36 females and 13 males) were treated surgically for a haemangioma of the liver in our clinic (own unpublished data). The majority of patients were aged between 20 and 40 years. 55% of the patients presented for diagnostics due to pain, in 45% of the cases the tumours were detected accidentally during examinations for other complaints.

In 36 patients the tumours had a diameter of 10 – 20 cm. The surgical procedures performed were enucleation (n=27), atypical liver resection (n=7), segmental resection (n=5) and anatomical left or right hemihepatectomy (n=10). Due to postoperative secondary haemorrhage 2 of 49 patients required revision.

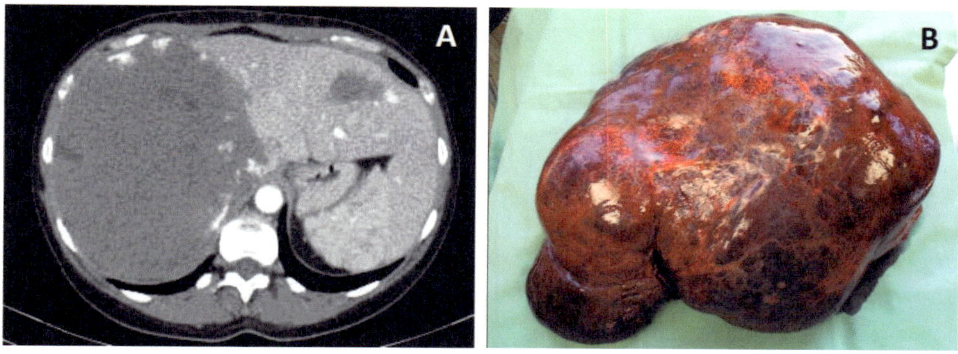

Figure 8. CT scan (**A**) and surgical specimen (**B**) of a large haemangioma of the liver.

3.9. Focal nodular hyperplasia

Hepatic FNH, a benign liver tumour, occurs approximately twice as frequently as hepatocellular adenoma. It is a disease affecting young, predominantly female adults (85%) with an incidence among the population of 20 per 100,000. In 15% of cases FNH can also be observed in mainly young adult males. As FNH predominantly occurs in females, the use of oral contraceptives is controversially suspected(Weimann et al.). Contrary to liver adenomas there is no description in the literature of malignant transformation. Without knowledge of the radiological findings it is often difficult to histologically confirm FNH due to the histologically normal, but enlarged structure of the hepatocytes. Vascular proliferation is evident, but is also observed for hepatic adenoma. Bile duct proliferation, on the other hand, is only evident in FNH. Both hepatic adenomas and FNH become symptomatic due to an increase in size and the subsequent compression and displacement of blood vessels and neighbouring organs. Apart from US, MR and CT can be used as diagnostic methods (Figure 9).

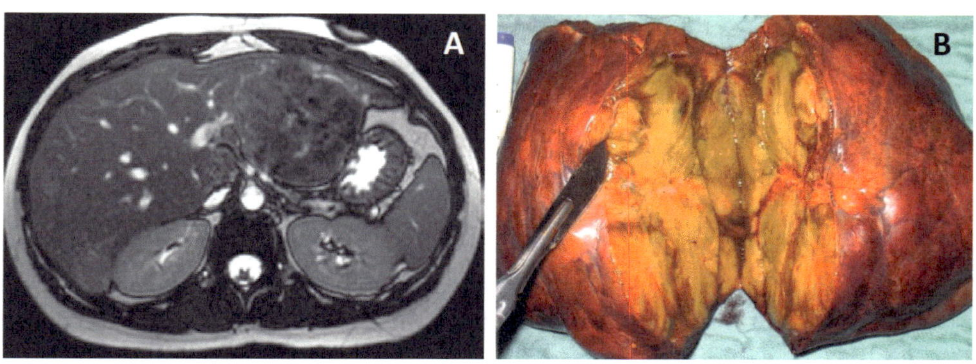

Figure 9. MRI scan (**A**) and surgical specimen (**B**) of a focal nodular hyperplasisa (FNH).

In approximately 95% of cases a hepatobiliary sequential scintiscanning can positively differentiate between FNH and hepatic adenoma. A definite sign is the central scar with its typical wheel spoke structure visible in the radiological image. Surgical intervention is only indicated when FNH becomes symptomatic. However, there are also cases when the explicit wish of a patient may be the indication for surgery. In these cases it is vital to inform the patient in detail of the possible risks and complications and the surgeon should seriously consider the possibility of carcinophobia.

In our opinion enucleation is the therapy of choice. Should this not be an option, the tumour can also be removed by either anatomical or atypical liver resection.

4. Special aspects of preoperative detailed information and informed consent

It is obvious that the patient prior to liver resection has to be informed in detail about risks generally involved in surgery, but also about those special complications usually associated with a liver resection (e.g. haemorrhage, secondary haemorrhage, thrombosis, pulmonary embolism, wound infection, injury of neighbouring organs). There is also the possibility of bile leakage, haemobilia, development of pleural effusion, icterus, chronic or acute hepatic insufficiency, pneumatohemia, acute pancreatitis as well as thrombosis of the portal vein or the liver artery.

In most cases of liver resection it is either imperative or advisable to also remove the gallbladder at the same time. The reason for this is that when performing an anatomical left or right hemihepatectomy the gallbladder is either directly at the designated resection site or during a segmental or typical liver resection denervation and/or devascularisation of the gallbladder may result. Furthermore, it may be advisable to simultaneously remove the gallbladder to prevent future occurrence of cholecystolithiasis. Subsequently this would at some stage require a cholecystectomy and adhesions at the operation site obviously present a higher operation risk. Therefore, it is advisable to inform the patient also of a simultaneous cholecystectomy prior to the planned liver resection. This is a point that is easily forgotten when informing the patient about the risks of the forthcoming liver resection as the gallbladder is not the primary surgical target.

During the preoperative informative discussion about the liver resection it should also be pointed out that intra- or postoperatively a blood transfusion may be necessary. Despite the present stringent and very safe quality controls, a residual risk of transmission of a viral or bacterial infectious disease cannot be completely excluded. In spite of today's safe determination of the blood group and bedside tests performed, there are rare cases of transfusion of blood group incompatible blood products resulting in serious transfusion incident. The patient should also be informed of the possible use of local hemostyptics (e.g. fibrin sealant) containing heterologous proteins, which may also transmit an infection.

Neither should it remain unmentioned that after surgery the patient should refrain completely from taking any hepatotoxic substances (e.g. alcohol), at least during the several months lasting postoperative liver regeneration period.

5. Preparation for surgery

We would summarize the obligatory specific preparation for surgery as follows: laboratory (CHE, Quick, PTT, aminotransferase, bilirubin; blood count, coagulation, determination of blood group), assurance of sufficient provisioning of erythrocyte concentrates by the blood bank, CT or MRI images to plan the extent of resection, in case of cystic tumours echinoccoccus serology, existence of a written valid and adequate informed consent for the operation and anaesthesia by the patient. Depending on comorbidity and age of the patient additional investigations should be performed preoperatively, e.g. ECG, lung function test, endurance ECG and chest X-ray. When indicated one should also aim to consult the anaesthetist to assess the operational risk, and depending on the finding to consult the specialists for internal medicine to optimize the therapy of any comorbidity to minimize the risks prior to commencing surgery.

Furthermore, the cause for preoperatively elevated aminotransferases and/or evident impairment of the liver function categorically requires clarification in cooperation with an experienced hepatologist.

We believe that a 3-dimensional reconstruction of the hepatic vascular anatomy based on the individual digital CT data set is generally not absolutely necessary. It should be reserved for planning the operation of specific cases, for instance when the localization of the hepatic tumour is unfavourable, e.g. in direct proximity to the liver hilus or at confluence of right, central and left hepatic vein close to the confluence into the caval vein. In such cases this will enable the surgeon to decide whether an ex situ or ante situ resection to fully remove the tumour may be required or if primarily liver transplantation is the only option.

6. Anaesthesiological aspects

During liver resection the central venous pressure should not be too high as this would have a negative impact on the extent of bleeding from the resection area. Neither should the central venous pressure be too low when transecting hepatic veins and/or the caval vein as this would increase unnecessarily the risk of possible aeroembolism during the operation. This requires constructive cooperation with the anaesthetists. Therefore, during the liver resection the positive endexspiratory pressure (PEEP) should be around 8-9 mmHg and the amount of volume given should be in accordance with the measured central venous pressure. If possible, the anaesthesist should refrain from using potentially hepatotoxic medication to avoid increasing unnecessarily the risk of postoperative failure of the remaining liver.

7. Surgical techniques

It is vital for each liver resection to know in detail the functional anatomy of the liver, i.e. the definition of the hemodynamically independent parenchymal areas according to the Couinaud classification is an indispensible prerequisite for any surgeon performing a liver resection. The complete resection of functionally autonomous parenchymal areas perfused by one appending pedicle (branch supplying portal vein, hepatic artery and common hepatic duct) is termed anatomical resection. Here one distinguishes between sector orientated resections (e.g. right and left hemihepatectomy, left lateral liver resection of segments II and III, trisegmentectomy) and segment orientated resections (mono-, bi- and polysegmentectomy). Principally, a combination of different anatomical resections is often possible. This option should always be taken considered instead of extended resections, which are often associated with a greater loss of healthy liver tissue. On the other hand, even when choosing a combination, extending the parenchymal area to be dissected can increase the potential rate of complications (e.g. secondary haemorrhage, biliary fistula and necrosis of the wound lip). Extended resections transcend the anatomical en-bloc resection of segments II, III, IVa and IVb of a left hemihepatectomy (when necessary also including segment I). When extending the anatomical en-bloc resection of segments V, VI, VII and VIII, additional segments and/or the hepatic bifurcation and/or a cuff of the portal or the caval vein can also be resected. When performing a so called atypical resection the surgeon does not adhere to the anatomical segmentation of the liver. The reason for this is the aim to minimize the loss of functional liver tissue. An example is the enucleation of a hepatic haemangioma or FNH without safety margin or the atypical resection at different parts of the liver when resecting with a safety margin more than one liver metastasis. Depending on the individual situation, anatomical and atypical liver resections can be combined. A special technique is the analogue ex situ resection (i.e. outside the patient's body) of the liver. The liver is then perfused with a conservation solution (e.g. HTK) and cooled to ensure the organ survives the ischaemic time until autotransplantation. Another rare resection technique is the ante situ resection. In this case the liver is dislocated from caudal to cranial in front of the abdomen after the complete hilus and the infrahepatic caval vein have been dissected, and after perfusion with a conservation solution (e.g. HTK) and cooling analogue to an organ to be transplanted. Finally, the liver hilus and continuity of the clamped and dissected infrahepatic caval vein have to be reconstructed by anastomoses. However, this technique obviously requires a surgeon with adequate specific surgical experience in the field of liver transplantation.

7.1. Methods to control haemorrhages

During preparation close to the large hepatic veins and the caval vein aeroembolism and severe bleeding can occur should these veins be injured. Severe bleeding can cause considerable obstruction of vision and endanger systematic and safe anastomosing of the blood vessels. To avoid such a situation it is necessary to have a clear view of the suprahepatic and infrahepatic caval vein. This ensures that, when needed, the vessel can be manually compressed and if necessary vascular clamps applied for safe closure by controlled suture of a large lesion without unnecessary constriction of these veins. Far reaching sutures performed with large needles, when the vision is impaired due to a large pool of blood, can have catastrophic sequelae, and such situations may easily occur to surgeons lacking the required evidence to perform larger liver resections. Larger haemorrhages at the resection area caused by dissection of large hepatic veins or branches of the portal vein or the hepatic artery can be safely controlled by manual compression of the residual liver lobe. If this is insufficient due to the extent of the haemorrhage, the surgeon additionally can use the Pringle manoeuvre with temporary occlusion of the liver hilus and if necessary additional clamping of the supra- and infrahepatic caval vein. To ensure that this possible, the preparatory precondition prior to dissecting the parenchyma is provision of the appropriate vessel loop at the liver hilus in the region of the hepatoduodenale ligament and at the infrahepatic caval vein. Should, in spite of all safety measures, an uncontrollable haemorrhage still occur, according to the current state of surgical knowledge a treatment error can be assumed. In the worst case, one has to consider that often the temporary haemostasis by packing with an abdominal pad is the best strategy, as one would do in case of a central liver trauma with massive haemorrhage and typical poor surgical vision. However, to ensure effective haemostasis it is necessary to completely mobilise the liver into a position that permits compression of the liver with abdominal pads from all sides. After stabilisation and when indicated, transfer of the patient to a centre for hepatobiliary surgery, where these pads can be removed and the haemorrhage finally stopped in a second-look-operation. In such situations it is again vital to avoid deep sutures with a large needle as this would evoke the danger to compromise vital central structures (e.g. portal vein, hepatic artery and/or central bile duct).

In current studies it could be shown that there are significant differences with respect to morbidity or mortality regarding the application of Pringle manoeuvre and selective, total or modified vascular occlusion (Ishizuka et al.).

7.2. Prevention of postoperative problems

Particularly when performing a right hemihepatectomy or an extended right hemihepatectomy the surgeon should fixate the remaining liver lobe with a suture, i.e. reattach the remaining falciform ligament to the abdominal wall in order to avoid kinking of the portal vein with subsequent thrombosis. In case of the anatomical right hemihepatectomy, as well as the anatomical left hepatectomy, the surgeon should bear in mind the need to prevent iatrogenic stenosis of the portal vein. This can be achieved by ensuring that the distance been the branch of the portal vein and the branch that remains is great enough without causing an unnecessary constriction, e.g. hour glass stenosis.

7.3. Methods of parenchyma dissection

A systematic meta-analysis of the various techniques for dissection of the parenchyma could not identify any differences between CUSA, radiofrequency sealer and hydrojet when compared to the conventional clamp crushing. It is important during liver resection that haemostasis at the resection surface is adequate, and it is equally important to take adequate care of the dissected bile ducts during a liver resection, e.g. titanium clips. We believe that suturing larger bile ducts is the safer method, however, stringent attention has to be paid to prevent accidental closure of the larger bile ducts of the remaining liver lobe. In a prospective, randomised study including 300 patients it could be demonstrated that the use of fibrin sealant on the resection area did not reduce blood loss, number of blood transfusions required, frequency of bile leaks, and neither did it improve the result of the resection. Therefore, considering also the cost we do not routinely apply fibrin sealant at our clinic.

7.4. Intraoperative US

Today, the use of intraoperative US is frequently used as standard procedure during liver resection to intraoperatively define exactly the resection margins and to detect possible additional masses in the liver. Should the histology report describe a margin forming malignant tumour, one has to consider at least that the tumour resection was microscopically incomplete. If in such a case no additional resection and no intraoperative US have been performed, it can be assumed that without detailed information the surgeon incorrectly assessed and defined the intrahepatic extension of the tumour and did not follow-up consequentially with further resection. However, in case of critical resections, when a postoperative failure of the small-sized residual liver has to be feared, it may be unavoidable to refrain from further extending the resection and/or it has to be accepted that an incomplete resection is inevitable. In such cases it is relevant that this deliberation is described and documented in the operation report to ensure that no treatment error (e.g. unnecessarily insufficiently radical oncologic resection) can be insinuated.

7.5. Laparoscopic liver surgery

During an international consensus conference on laparoscopic liver surgery held in Kentucky with 45 international experts from continents participating, the indication, patient selection, surgical techniques, complications and patient safety as well as further relevant surgical education aspects of laparoscopic liver surgery were specifically discussed (Buell, J. F et al). Hereby laparoscopic liver surgery included per definition solely the laparoscopic method (hand-assisted laparoscopic approach and hybrid technique). Mutual consent was reached on the point that this technique could be applied in patients with solitary liver lesions (<5 cm) in segments II – VI. The participants of this consensus conference agreed that already today the left lateral laparoscopic segmentectomy (liver segments II and III) should be considered the standard procedure compared with the open surgical technique. Concerning all forms of liver resection, including anatomical right and left hemihepatectomy, it was the opinion of the consensus conference that these types of laparoscopic liver resections should only be performed by particularly experienced surgeons who are sufficiently familiar with the more advanced extended openliver resections. The indication for conversion from laparoscopic to open surgical technique should be considered liberally in case of technically difficult, time-consuming resections and congruent aspects of patient safety. One should always attempt to initially control complications caused by haemorrhages laparoscopically before conversing to the open surgical approach. Using the combination of hand-assisted laparoscopic technique and the hybrid method may be quicker and more effective than the purely laparoscopic method. In case of benign liver lesions the indication for surgery should not just be considered

http://dx.doi.org/10.5772/55932

because one can operate laparoscopically. For transplantation in children, the purely laparoscopic approach has already been used for the donation of the left lateral liver lobe (segment II and III), whereas for living donation for adult recipients only the hand-assisted laparoscopic procedure has been used so far. So far, safety and efficacy of laparoscopic liver resection have not been adequately analysed, particularly not in controlled studies comparing laparoscopic and open surgical techniques. Currently, it appears that a prospective randomised study cannot be realised due to logistic problems. However, there is agreement on the subject of initiating an international registry to document the role and safety of laparoscopic liver resection.

8. Postoperative treatment

In case of a rapid and unexpected postoperative rise of the liver enzymes (e.g. AST, ALT), a sudden thrombosis of the portal vein should be considered. Such prevalent complications occurring after liver resection are not necessarily evidence of a treatment error. However, it is important that these complications, if they occur, are not overlooked and that a quick and effective therapy is initiated. If a sudden postoperative elevation of aminotransferases occurs, the possibility of a thrombosis has to be considered and a Doppler-US and/or CT with i.v. contrast medium during the arterial and porta-venous phase should be initiated immediately. Evidence of a thrombosed portal vein requires the immediate performance of an emergency thrombectomy followed by PTT-effective heparinisation.

Particularly bilious peritonitis is a complication that should not be underestimated, even with good drainage. When in doubt as in the absence of distinct clinical improvement or in spite of CT- or US-guided placement of a system to drain the bilioma, the indication for a revision should be considered rather liberally.

Early mobilisation and adequate respiratory training should also not be underestimated as effective methods to prevent pulmonary and thrombo-embolic complications.

Early contact with a liver transplantation centre is recommended should failure of the residual liver occur. Generally, such a centre not only has the ability to perform transplantation, but often clinical experimental methods to assist the liver function are available.

Author details

H. Bektas*, H. Schrem, M. Kleine, A. Tamac, F.W.R. Vondran, S. Uzunyayla and J. Klempnauer

*Address all correspondence to: Bektas.Hueseyin@mh-hannover.de

Allgemein-, Viszeral- und Transplantationschirurgie, Medizinische Hochschule Hannover, Germany

References

[1] Becker, T, Lehner, F, Bektas, H, Lueck, R, Nashan, B, & Klempnauer, J. . (2001). [Stellenwert der Lebertransplantation beim hepatocellulären Karzinom.]. *Der Onkologe* 12, 1296-1304.

[2] Bektas, H, Lehner, F, Werner, U, Bartels, M, Piso, P, Tusch, G, Schrem, H, & Klempnauer, J. (2001). Surgical therapy of cystic echinococcosis of the liver]. *Zentralbl Chir* 126, (5), 369-373.

[3] Bektas, H, Schrem, H, Kleine, M, Laenger, F, Lehner, F, Kaaden, S, Becker, T, & Klempnauer, J. (2010). Chirurgische Intervention beim Leberrundherd. Indikation und Verfahren.]. *Chir. Praxis* , 72, 39-58.

[4] Bhangui, P, Vibert, E, Majno, P, Salloum, C, Andreani, P, Zocrato, J, Ichai, P, Saliba, F, Adam, R, Castaing, D, & Azoulay, D. (2011). Intention-to-treat analysis of liver transplantation for hepatocellular carcinoma: living versus deceased donor transplantation. *Hepatology* 53, (5), 1570-1579.

[5] Bioulac-sage, P, Laumonier, H, Laurent, C, Zucman-rossi, J, & Balabaud, C. (2008). Hepatocellular adenoma: what is new in 2008. *Hepatol Int* 2, (3), 316-321.

[6] Boozari, B, Lotz, J, Galanski, M, & Gebel, M. (2007). Diagnostic imaging of liver tumours. Current status]. *Internist (Berl)* 48, (1), 8, 10-12, 14-16, 18-20.

[7] Bosch, F. X, Ribes, J, Diaz, M, & Cleries, R. (2004). Primary liver cancer: worldwide incidence and trends. *Gastroenterology* 127, (5 Suppl 1), SS16., 5.

[8] Breitenstein, S, Dimitroulis, D, Petrowsky, H, Puhan, M. A, Mullhaupt, B, & Clavien, P. A. (2009). Systematic review and meta-analysis of interferon after curative treatment of hepatocellular carcinoma in patients with viral hepatitis. *Br J Surg* 96, (9), 975-981.

[9] Bruix, J, Sherman, M, Llovet, J. M, Beaugrand, M, Lencioni, R, Burroughs, A. K, Christensen, E, Pagliaro, L, Colombo, M, & Rodes, J. (2001). Clinical management of hepatocellular carcinoma. Conclusions of the Barcelona-2000 EASL conference. European Association for the Study of the Liver. *J Hepatol* 35, (3), 421-430.

[10] Buell, J. F, Cherqui, D, Geller, D. A, Rourke, O, Iannitti, N, Dagher, D, Koffron, I, Thomas, A. J, Gayet, M, Han, B, Wakabayashi, H. S, Belli, G, Kaneko, G, Ker, H, Scatton, C. G, Laurent, O, Abdalla, A, Chaudhury, E. K, Dutson, P, Gamblin, E, Angelica, C. , D, Nagorney, M, Testa, D, Labow, G, Manas, D, Poon, D, Nelson, R. T, Martin, H, Clary, R, Pinson, B, Martinie, W. C, Vauthey, J, Goldstein, J. N, Roayaie, R, Barlet, S, Espat, D, Abecassis, J, Rees, M, Fong, M, Mcmasters, Y, Broelsch, K. M, Busuttil, C, Belghiti, R, Strasberg, J, & Chari, S. R. S. ((2009). The international position on laparoscopic liver surgery: The Louisville Statement, 2008. *Ann Surg* 250, (5), 825-830.

[11] Czermak, B. V, Akhan, O, Hiemetzberger, R, Zelger, B, Vogel, W, Jaschke, W, Rieger, M, Kim, S. Y, & Lim, J. H. (2008). Echinococcosis of the liver. *Abdom Imaging* 33, (2), 133-143.

[12] Deneve, J. L, Pawlik, T. M, Cunningham, S, Clary, B, Reddy, S, Scoggins, C. R, Martin, R. C, Angelica, D, Staley, M, Choti, C. A, Jarnagin, M. A, Schulick, W. R, & Kooby, R. D. D. A. ((2009). Liver cell adenoma: a multicenter analysis of risk factors for rupture and malignancy. *Ann Surg Oncol* 16, (3), 640-648.

[13] DuBrayB. J., Jr., Chapman, W. C. & Anderson, C. D. ((2011). Hepatocellular carcinoma: a review of the surgical approaches to management. *Mo Med* 108, (3), 195-198.

[14] EASL-EORTC Clinical Practice Guidelines: Management of hepatocellular carcinomaJournal of Hepatology (2012). j 908-943, 56

[15] Figueras, J, Llado, L, Miro, M, Ramos, E, Torras, J, Fabregat, J, & Serrano, T. (2007).

[16] Application of fibrin glue sealant after hepatectomy does not seem justified: results of a randomized study in 300 patients*Ann Surg* 245, (4), 536-542.

[17] Galanski, M, Jordens, S, & Weidemann, J. (2008). Diagnosis and differential diagnosis of benign liver tumors and tumor-like lesions]. *Chirurg* 79, (8), 707-721.

[18] Gratz, K. F, & Weimann, A. (1998). Diagnosis of liver tumors--when is scintigraphy of value?]. *Zentralbl Chir* 123, (2), 111-118.

[19] Greten, T. F, Papendorf, F, Bleck, J. S, Kirchhoff, T, Wohlberedt, T, Kubicka, S, Klempnauer, J, Galanski, M, & Manns, M. P. (2005). Survival rate in patients with hepatocellular carcinoma: a retrospective analysis of 389 patients. *Br J Cancer* 92, (10), 1862-1868.

[20] Guiteau, J. J, Cotton, R. T, Karpen, S. J, Mahony, O, & Goss, C. A. J. A. ((2010). Pediatric liver transplantation for primary malignant liver tumors with a focus on hepatic epithelioid hemangioendothelioma: the UNOS experience. *Pediatr Transplant* 14, (3), 326-331.

[21] Hamelmann, H, & Grabiger, A. (1968). Hepatic echinococcus. Diagnosis and therapy]. *Munch Med Wochenschr* 110, (8), 441-445.

[22] Ishikawa, T. (2010). Clinical features of hepatitis B virus-related hepatocellular carcinoma. *World J Gastroenterol* 16, (20), 2463-2467.

[23] Ishizuka, M, Kubota, K, Kita, J, Shimoda, M, Kato, M, & Sawada, T. (2011). Duration of hepatic vascular inflow clamping and survival after liver resection for hepatocellular carcinoma. *Br J Surg* 98, (9), 1284-1290.

[24] Kirchhoff, T. D, Bleck, J. S, Dettmer, A, Chavan, A, Rosenthal, H, Merkesdal, S, Frericks, B, Zender, L, Malek, N. P, Greten, T. F, Kubicka, S, Manns, M. P, & Galanski, M. (2007). Transarterial chemoembolization using degradable starch microspheres and

iodized oil in the treatment of advanced hepatocellular carcinoma: evaluation of tumor response, toxicity, and survival. *Hepatobiliary Pancreat Dis Int* 6, (3), 259-266.

[25] Klatskin, G. (1977). Hepatic tumors: possible relationship to use of oral contraceptives. *Gastroenterology* 73, (2), 386-394.

[26] Kleine, M, Schrem, H, Vondran, F, Krech, T, Klempnauer, J, & Bektas, H. (2011). Extended surgery in advanced pancreatic endocrine tumours. *BJS* in press.

[27] Kornprat, P, Cerwenka, H, Bacher, H, Shabrawi, A, Tillich, M, Langner, C, & Mischinger, H. J. (2004). Minimally invasive management of dysontogenetic hepatic cysts. *Langenbecks Arch Surg* 389, (4), 289-292.

[28] Kulik, U, Framke, T, Grosshennig, A, Ceylan, A, Bektas, H, Klempnauer, J, & Lehner, F. (2011). Liver Resection of Colorectal Liver Metastases in Elderly Patients. *World J Surg* 35, (9), 2063-2072.

[29] Lang, H, & Broelsch, C. E. (2007). Liver resection and transplantation for hepatic tumors]. *Internist (Berl)* 48, (1), 30-39.

[30] Llovet, J. M, Ricci, S, Mazzaferro, V, Hilgard, P, Gane, E, Blanc, J. F, De Oliveira, A. C, Santoro, A, Raoul, J. L, Forner, A, Schwartz, M, Porta, C, Zeuzem, S, Bolondi, L, Greten, T. F, Galle, P. R, Seitz, J. F, Borbath, I, Haussinger, D, Giannaris, T, Shan, M, Moscovici, M, Voliotis, D, & Bruix, J. (2008). Sorafenib in advanced hepatocellular carcinoma. *N Engl J Med* 359, (4), 378-390.

[31] Lochan, R, White, S. A, & Manas, D. M. (2007). Liver resection for colorectal liver metastasis. *Surg Oncol* 16, (1), 33-45.

[32] Malhi, H, & Gores, G. J. (2006). Cholangiocarcinoma: modern advances in understanding a deadly old disease. *J Hepatol* 45, (6), 856-867.

[33] Marelli, L, Stigliano, R, Triantos, C, Senzolo, M, Cholongitas, E, Davies, N, Tibballs, J, Meyer, T, Patch, D. W, & Burroughs, A. K. (2007). Transarterial therapy for hepatocellular carcinoma: which technique is more effective? A systematic review of cohort and randomized studies. *Cardiovasc Intervent Radiol* 30, (1), 6-25.

[34] Marrero, J. A, Fontana, R. J, Fu, S, Conjeevaram, H. S, Su, G. L, & Lok, A. S. (2005). Alcohol, tobacco and obesity are synergistic risk factors for hepatocellular carcinoma. *J Hepatol* 42, (2), 218-224.

[35] Mehrabi, A, Kashfi, A, Fonouni, H, Schemmer, P, Schmied, B. M, Hallscheidt, P, Schirmacher, P, Weitz, J, Friess, H, Buchler, M. W, & Schmidt, J. (2006). Primary malignant hepatic epithelioid hemangioendothelioma: a comprehensive review of the literature with emphasis on the surgical therapy. *Cancer* 107, (9), 2108-2121.

[36] Mohr, L. (2007). Hepatocellular carcinoma: novel therapeutic approaches]. *Praxis (Bern 1994)* 96, (14), 553-562.

[37] Moreno GonzalezE., Rico Selas, P., Martinez, B., Garcia Garcia, I., Palma Carazo, F. & Hidalgo Pascual, M. ((1991). Results of surgical treatment of hepatic hydatidosis: current therapeutic modifications. *World J Surg* 15, (2), 254-263.

[38] Nichols, J. C, & Gores, G. J. LaRusso, N. F., Wiesner, R. H., Nagorney, D. M. & Ritts, R. E., Jr. ((1993). Diagnostic role of serum CA for cholangiocarcinoma in patients with primary sclerosing cholangitis. *Mayo Clin Proc* 68, (9), 874-879., 19-9.

[39] Pamecha, V, Gurusamy, K. S, Sharma, D, & Davidson, B. R. (2009). Techniques for liver parenchymal transection: a meta-analysis of randomized controlled trials. *HPB (Oxford)* 11, (4), 275-281.

[40] Pawlik, T. M, & Choti, M. A. (2007). Surgical therapy for colorectal metastases to the liver. *J Gastrointest Surg* 11, (8), 1057-1077.

[41] Rooks, J. B, Ory, H. W, Ishak, K. G, Strauss, L. T, Greenspan, J. R, Hill, A. P, & Tyler, C. W. Jr. ((1979). Epidemiology of hepatocellular adenoma. The role of oral contraceptive use. *JAMA* 242, (7), 644-648.

[42] Ros, P. R, & Li, K. C. (1989). Benign liver tumors. *Curr Probl Diagn Radiol* 18, (3), 125-155.

[43] Scatton, O, Zalinski, S, Jegou, D, Compagnon, P, Lesurtel, M, Belghiti, J, Boudjema, K, Lentschener, C, & Soubrane, O. (2011). Randomized clinical trial of ischaemic preconditioning in major liver resection with intermittent Pringle manoeuvre. *Br J Surg* 98, (9), 1236-1243.

[44] Schrem, H, Bektas, H, & Klempnauer, J. (2004). Hepatobiliäre und pankreatische Chirurgie.]. *Jahrbuch der Chirurgie*.

[45] Shaib, Y. H, Serag, H. B, Nooka, A. K, Thomas, M, Brown, T. D, Patt, Y. Z, & Hassan, M. M. Risk factors for intrahepatic and extrahepatic cholangiocarcinoma: a hospital-based case-control study. Am J Gastroenterol (2007). May;, 102(5), 1016-1021.

[46] Shi, M, Guo, R. P, Lin, X. J, Zhang, Y. Q, Chen, M. S, Zhang, C. Q, Lau, W. Y, & Li, J. Q. (2007). Partial hepatectomy with wide versus narrow resection margin for solitary hepatocellular carcinoma: a prospective randomized trial. *Ann Surg* 245, (1), 36-43.

[47] Singal, A. K, Vauthey, J. N, Grady, J. J, & Stroehlein, J. R. (2011). Intra-hepatic cholangiocarcinoma--frequency and demographic patterns: thirty-year data from the M.D. Anderson Cancer Center. *J Cancer Res Clin Oncol* 137, (7), 1071-1078.

[48] Spangenberg, H. C, Thimme, R, & Blum, H. E. (2006). Serum markers of hepatocellular carcinoma. *Semin Liver Dis* 26, (4), 385-390.

[49] Spangenberg, H. C, Thimme, R, & Blum, H. E. (2007). Liver Masses. *Dtsch Arztebl International* 104, (33), 2279-.

[50] Spangenberg, H. C, Thimme, R, Mohr, L, & Blum, H. E. (2007). The hepatocellular carcinoma: alternative therapeutical strategies]. *Zentralbl Chir* 132, (4), 322-327.

[51] Strey, C, Zapletal, C, & Bechstein, W. (2007). Surgical therapy of hepatocellular carcinoma. *Der Gastroenterologe*.

[52] Wanless, I. R, Mawdsley, C, & Adams, R. (1985). On the pathogenesis of focal nodular hyperplasia of the liver. *Hepatology* 5, (6), 1194-1200.

[53] Weimann, A, Ringe, B, Klempnauer, J, Lamesch, P, Gratz, K. F, Prokop, M, Maschek, H, Tusch, G, & Pichlmayr, R. (1997). Benign liver tumors: differential diagnosis and indications for surgery. *World J Surg* 21, (9), 983-990; discussion , 990-981.

[54] Wilkens, L, Bredt, M, Flemming, P, Becker, T, Klempnauer, J, & Kreipe, H. H. (2001). Differentiation of liver cell adenomas from well-differentiated hepatocellular carcinomas by comparative genomic hybridization. *J Pathol* 193, (4), 476-482.

Chapter 6

Post-Therapeutic Follow-Up and Early Detection of Recurrence in Hepatocellular Carcinoma

Simona Ioanițescu, L. Micu, Mariana Mihăilă and
R. Badea

Additional information is available at the end of the chapter

http://dx.doi.org/10.5772/55778

1. Introduction

Hepatocellular carcinoma (HCC) represents the fifth cause of death due to cancer in the world. Approximately half a million new cases are recorded globally each year [1,2].

The most important risk factors include chronic infection with hepatitis B or hepatitis C viruses, alcoholic liver disease and nonalcoholic fatty liver disease. Less frequent causes of HCC are haemochromatosis, Wilson's disease and autoimmune hepatitis.

The early diagnosis of HCC relies on careful follow-up of patients with increased risk of developing the disease, in accordance with the AASLD and EASL-EORTC guidelines from 2010 and 2012, respectively.

Current treatment of HCC is based on the updated Barcelona algorithm [3]. According to this algorithm, therapeutic options for HCC are divided into curative treatments (resection, liver transplantation and radiofrequency/percutaneous ethanol injection) for HCC in very early stage or early stage (A), transarterial chemoembolization (TACE) for intermediate stage (B) HCC, sorafenib for advanced stage (C) HCC and best supportive care for terminal stage (D) HCC. The following therapies should be applied depending on the stage of HCC:

- stage 0 (PST 0, Child-Pugh A) represents very early stage (0) HCC, with a single tumor < 2 cm or carcinoma *in situ*. When portal pressure/bilirubin are normal, resection is indicated. In case portal pressure/bilirubin are increased, liver transplantation is the therapy of choice in the absence of important comorbidities, or RFA in case of associated diseases.
- Stage A-C (PST 0-2, Child-Pugh A-B) is classified into early stage (A) (single or 3 nodules ≤ 3 cm, PS 0), intermediate stage (B) (multinodular, PS 0) and advanced stage (C) (Portal

invasion, N1, M1, PS 1-2). For early stage (A) HCC, in case of a single nodule the same algorithm applies as for very early stage (0) HCC; in case of 3 nodules ≤ 3 cm, liver transplantation or RFA should be performed, depending on the absence or presence of associated diseases. For intermediate stage (B) HCC transarterial chemoembolization (TACE) is advised, while for advanced stage (C) HCC sorafenib is indicated.

- Stage D (PST > 2, Child-Pugh C) represents terminal stage (D) and only benefits from best supportive care [3].
- Currently, the 5-year survival rate after surgical resection and transplant is of 70-80%, and of 70% after local ablative procedures [4-7].

The post-therapeutic follow-up and early detection of recurrences represent an important problem in the management of patients with HCC.

2. Definition of therapeutic response to therapy and methods for its evaluation

HCC presents several therapeutic peculiarities that must be taken into account when monitoring therapy. Studies have shown that HCC is associated in over 90% of cases with chronic liver disease of viral etiology [8]. In approximately 80% of cases the tumor develops in a previously cirrhotic liver, characterized by disruption of the lobular architecture of the liver and nodular reorganization of the hepatic parenchyma [9]. Malignant transformation is more frequent in cirrhotic livers, with a frequency of 80-90% being noted in autopsy-based studies [10, 11], while 59-94% of newly diagnosed nodules in cirrhosis are histologically proven to be malignant [11-13].

Carcinogenesis is a multistep and multicentric process, the evolution from regenerative nodule to dysplastic nodule to HCC taking place in different phases of the progression of liver cirrhosis; therefore it is possible to simultaneously present regenerative nodules, nodules with different degrees of dysplasia and even early-stage HCC, alongside a nodule or nodules already diagnosed as HCC. Changes in the intranodular vascularization lie at the heart of carcinogenesis, consisting in a chaotic and explosive development of arterial neovascularization with a gradual decrease to disappearance of portal vascularization [14]. Changes in intratumoral vascularization are specific to HCC and allow for its imaging-based diagnosis [15].

Treatment of HCC is complex, and according to the staging of the tumor, therapies can be radical or palliative, local, loco-regional or systemic.

Different criteria for evaluating efficiency of HCC therapy have been investigated over the years.

The first criteria used for monitoring oncological therapies were those based only on measurement of tumor dimensions, namely unidimensional – RECIST criteria (Response Evaluation Criteria in Solid Tumours), modified RECIST 1.1, and bidimensional – WHO (World Health

Organization) criteria. However it was later shown that the degree of necrosis induced by therapy does not necessarily correlate with tumoral dimensions, and measurement of only tumor diameters is not sufficient for evaluating response to therapy.

In 2001, the European Association for the Study of the Liver (EASL) introduced evaluation of tumoral necrosis induced by therapy as a criterion for assessing response to therapy, by using contrast-enhanced dynamic imaging techniques.

The American Association for the Study of Liver Diseases (AASLD) later endorsed this criterion and introduced it in the *AASLD practice guideline on the management of HCC*, published in 2005.

In 2008, a group of experts determined a series of additions and changes to the RECIST criteria, useful both in clinical practice and in complex studies of new targeted therapies. These ammendments were published in the „AASLD-JNCI (Journal of the National Cancer Institute) guideline" as the mRECIST (modified RECIST) criteria. These criteria have been endorsed and are currently recommended by the European Association for the Study of the Liver (EASL) and by the European Organization for Research and Treatment of Cancer (EORTC) in the first common guideline, "EASL-EORTC Clinical Practice Guidelines: Management of hepatocellular carcinoma" published in 2012.

According to these guidelines, post-therapeutic evaluation of patients with cirrhosis and HCC is based exclusively on contrast-enhanced dynamic imaging criteria. The recommended techniques are contrast-enhanced spiral CT scan or contrast-enhanced MRI. Other imaging techniques, such as angiography, contrast-enhanced ultrasound and PET-CT, are appreciated as "controversial" [3]. It is worth mentioning that their role is analyzed especially in positive diagnosis of HCC more than in post-therapeutic monitoring.

CT and MRI have the advantage of being easier to standardize. Ultrasonography, even using second-generation contrast media, remains an operator-dependent method and requires specialists with training and experience in this field.

CT scan allows for performing very thin slices. Standard practice is represented by successive slices with a thickness of 5 mm and a reconstruction interval of 5 mm, therefore making possible identification of lesions with a minimal diameter of 1 cm. The lesions are measured either in the arterial phase or in the portal-venous phase, when we have a maximal contrast from the normal parenchyma and when the margins of the lesion are clearly delineated [16].

The protocol for post-therapeutic monitoring includes a mandatory initial imaging examination less than 4 weeks before the start of treatment considered as a baseline exam. On this occasion the lesions are divided into measurable and non-measurable. Measurable lesions are lesions that can be correctly measured in at least one dimension, which are reproducible and measurable at later examinations, and that are larger than 1 cm. Target lesions are selected from these measurable lesions [16].

The RECIST 1.1 criteria evaluate therapeutic response by measuring the sum of the maximal diameters of the target lesion (in total 5 lesions, maximum 2 per organ), the remaining lesions being considered as non-target. A change compared to the RECIST criteria is the fact that enlarged lymph nodes are considered to be target, distinct from the hepatic target lesions and are considered pathological if the short axis is ≥ 15 mm. Lymph nodes ≥ 10 - < 15 mm are considered to be non-target, while lymph nodes < 10 mm non-pathological. Evaluation of global response in the RECIST 1.1 criteria include analysis both of target lesions and of non-target lesions [17].

Compared to the RECIST 1.1 criteria, the mRECIST criteria measure the maximum diameter of the viable segment (which captures contrast media) of the tumor. In order to be considered a target lesion, the hyperenhancing area must be measurable (at least 1 cm), clearly delineated and reproducible at later examinations.

It is important to note that infiltrative HCC must be considered as a non-target lesion when its contour is not well delineated and does not allow precise repeated measurements during further examinations. Furthermore, previously treated tumors can be considered as target lesions only if the intralesional hyperenhancing area is measurable, being clearly delineated, if it measures at least 1 cm and is reproducible at further examinations [16].

According to the mRECIST criteria adopted by EASL in the EASL-EORTC Practice Guidelines, the following definitions should be used:

- complete response (CR) for target lesions is defined as " disappearance of any intratumoral arterial enhancement in all target lesions";
- partial response (PR): "at least a 30% decrease in the sum of the diameters of viable (enhancement in the arterial phase) target lesions, taking as reference the baseline sum of the diameters of target lesions";
- stable disease (SD): "any case that does not qualify for either PR or PD";
- progressive disease (PD): "any increase of at least 20% in the sum of diameters of viable (enhancing) target lesions, taking as reference the smallest sum of the diameters of viable target lesions recorded since treatment started" [3].

In case of non-target lesions, the following definitions apply:

- CR represents "dissappearance of any intratumoral arterial enhancement in all non-target lesions";
- incomplete response (IR) or SD: "persistence of intratumoral arterial enhancement in one or more non-target lesions";
- PD: "appearance of one or more new lesions and/or unequivocal progression of existing non-target lesions" [3,16]

Moreover, the mRECIST criteria include a series of special recommendations related to portal vein thrombosis, periportal adenopathies, presence of pleural effusions and/or ascites. Thus, malignant thrombosis of the portal vein must be considered as a non-measurable lesion, due to the difficulties in providing an exact measurement and in later repeating the measurements. Periportal reactive lymph nodes are frequently encountered in viral liver disease. They are considered malignant only when the short axis of the lymph nodes measure more than 20 mm.

Ascites and pleural effusions rarely develop as complications in the evolution of HCC due to the fact that peritoneal carcinomatosis is rare, but appear frequently as markers of the worsening of liver cirrhosis. This is the reason for which experts insist, in the new mRECIST criteria, on cytohistological confirmation of the neoplastic nature of pleural effusions and especially of ascites when they appear or progress during treatment, and when the liver lesions do not meet the criteria for progressive disease [16; 18].

Another aspect that is analyzed is represented by defining hepatic lesions appearing during therapy or post-therapy as malignant and thus recording disease progression. The difficulty derives from the heterogenous and nodular aspect of the cirrhotic hepatic parenchyma, in which we can simultaneously encounter regenerative nodules and nodules with different degrees of dysplasia, as well as changes in the vascularization dynamics of these nodules during the process of carcinogenesis. All these details explain the difficulties in diagnosing early-stage HCC. Respecting the diagnostic criteria for HCC endorsed by the EASL and AASLD guidelines, experts have introduced the following recommendations related to disease progression in the mRECIST criteria:

- a newly discovered nodule is considered to be HCC if it measures over 1 cm and presents a vascular pattern typical for HCC;
- a nodule larger than 1 cm and with atypical vascular pattern is considered to be HCC if progression of its dimensions of at least 1 cm is recorded during further measurements;
- assessment of global therapeutic response takes into account target lesions, non-target lesions and development of new lesions. Any newly-discovered lesion with a pattern typical for HCC is considered to be a marker of disease progression regardless of the evolution of the target and non-target lesions. If the lesion has atypical features, it is considered to be unclear and inconclusive for recording disease progression at that time;
- disease progression can be recorded retrospectively if a newly discovered nodule, which did not initially meet the diagnostic criteria for HCC, gains typical vascular aspects during evolution [16].

Monitoring of global therapeutic response and of disease progression has generated over time a series of controversies. The possibility for retrospectively analyzing newly discovered liver masses during disease evolution represents an important element that has been introduced in therapeutic guidelines. This element takes into account the particularities of the natural evolution of the disease.

Another problem underlined by the groups of experts addresses the difficulty of assessing therapeutic response to local and loco-regional therapies, as well as when it would be correct to record disease progression.

EASL-EORTC Clinical Practice Guidelines recommend that "Assessment of response in HCC should be based on the mRECIST criteria (recommendation 2B)", and "Dynamic CT or MRI are recommended tools to assess response one month after resection, loco-regional or systemic therapies (recommendation 1A)" [3].

The mRECIST criteria are useful in case of radiotherapy or systemic therapies, but are not as useful when treatment strictly addresses one mass or a group of masses, while the natural evolution of disease continues in the remaining hepatic parenchyma.

The Liver Cancer Study Group of Japan aimed to determine criteria for distinctly assessing local, loco-regional and systemic therapies - criteria which should be useful and applicable in clinical practice. The recommendations, known as RECICL (Response Evaluation Criteria in Cancer of the Liver), are applicable especially for local and loco-regional therapies (TACE), but also for radiotherapy or systemic therapies, in combination with the WHO and RECIST criteria. These criteria, first published in 1994, were revised and completed in 2004 and 2009.

The main concept of the 2004 RECICL (and the difference from the RECIST and WHO criteria) was the analysis only of the treated mass, excluding the appearance of new lesions from the assessment of the direct therapeutic effect on the previously treated lesion by local or loco-regional therapies. Experts affirm that in case of loco-regional therapies, the appearance of new intrahepatic lesions in another area than that subjected to treatment should not necessarily be considered as progressive disease. However, in global evaluation, the appearance of new lesions is regarded as progressive disease, and new lesions are described separately [19].

The evaluation criteria are mainly imaging based, including both dimensional variations of the tumor and the assessment of the therapeutically induced degree of necrosis. The Japanese experts consider that measurement of tumoral dimensions in two axes (the first being the maximum diameter of the tumor and the second being perpendicular on the first) is more exact than measuring only the maximum diameter of the tumor, as is recommended by the RECIST criteria. A maximum of 5 target lesions are chosen for global evaluation of therapy when more than 5 lesions are present, but CR is defined as "100% tumor-necrotizing effect or 100% tumor size reduction rate" of all hepatic lesions, target or non-target, as opposed to the RECIST criteria, which define CR as " disappearance of all target lesions". In order to evaluate the direct therapeutic effect on the target lesion, each nodule is analyzed separately when multiple intrahepatic nodules are present [19].

The definitions of PR and PD also differ according to the criteria used for assessing response. Thus, RECICL regards PR as "tumor-necrotizing effect or tumor size reduction rate between 50% and < 100%", while the RECIST criteria define PR as "30% or greater reduction of target lesions". PD is defined in the RECICL criteria as "≥ 25% enlargement of the tumor regardless of the necrotizing effect or appearance of a new lesion", as opposed to the RECIST criteria where PD is considered a "≥ 20% increase or appearance of a new lesion" [19].

New lesions are classified by the Japanese authors into:

- intrahepatic solitary lesion (within or outside the treatment area);
- intrahepatic multiple lesions (within or outside the treatment area); or
- vascular invasion (the portal vein, hepatic vein, bile duct)/extrahepatic spread [19].

This classification was adopted in order to allow for a better appreciation of prognosis; thus, prognosis is more reserved when the new lesions are more disseminated.

http://dx.doi.org/10.5772/55778

It is important to note here the imaging aspects of CR, residual tumor and reccurence. The imaging of a complete therapeutic response is represented by the presence of non-enhanced areas on contrast examination which signify complete tumoral necrosis, with a safety rim around the tumor. In order to assess the efficiency of therapy, it is mandatory to compare the diameter of the tumor before therapy with that of the ablation zone. It is worth noting that in order to assess the CR of the treated nodule, the non-enhanced area must surpass or at least be equal to the tumoral dimensions, the two situations being classified separately (figure 1 a and b)[[19].

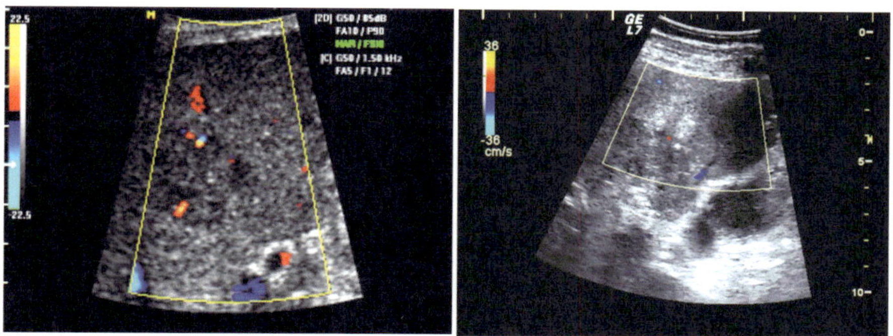

(a) (b)

Figure 1. a. HCC before therapy. 2D ultrasound and color Doppler examination. b. Same case, standard ultrasound and color Doppler examination after RFA. We remark that the dimensions of the post-RFA lesion are larger than the dimensions of the initial tumor.

In case of incomplete ablation, diameter of the tumor remains unchanged, and the residual tumoral tissue shows a non-regular outline and poorly delineated internal margins located at the periphery of the tumor. At contrast-enhanced CT or CEUS examinations its behavior is identical to that of the initial tumor (figure 2).

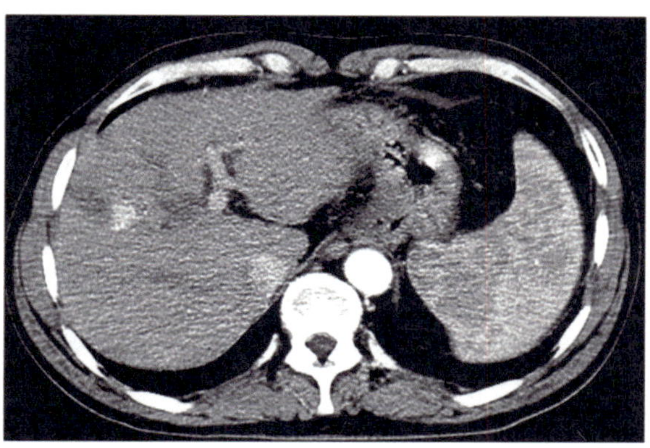

Figure 2. Partial response after RFA. CE-CT image, arterial phase. We remark residual tumoral tissue in the profound portion of the lesion.

Recurrences are defined as reappearance of intralesional areas at the tumor periphery with behaviour similar to HCC (hyperenhancing in the arterial phase and wash-out in the portal and parenchymal phases on contrast exams) at a certain time after the procedure. Especially in cases of HCC treated by percutaneous ethanol injection (PEI), the presence of hyperenhancing septa or vessels inside the tumor have been noted [20]. The increase of tumor size occurs later than changes in intralesional vascularization and serological markers; therefore early diagnosis of recurrences is based mainly on contrast-enhanced dynamic imaging examinations.

A new element also appears in assessing therapeutically-induced tumoral necrosis. It is known that post-TACE intralesional presence of lipiodol prevents contrast-enhanced examination of the nodule, especially the assessment of contrast enhancement of the lesion in the arterial phase. Lipiodol appears intensely hyperechoic at ultrasound examination with important posterior attenuation, which decreases visibility (figure 3).

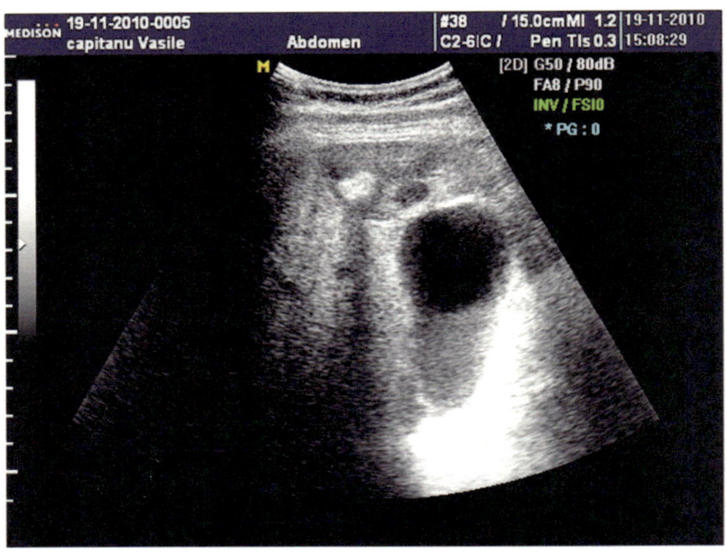

Figure 3. Baseline ultrasound examination 48 hours after TACE. Examination is hampered by the diffuse presence of lipiodol inside the liver. We remark lipiodol concentrated inside the lesion, intensely hyperechoic, with posterior shadow.

At CT examination lipiodol appears intensely hyperechoic inside the lesion, preventing contrast-enhanced examination. Lipiodol may persist months or even years inside the lesion (figure 4a and b). Studies have histologically demonstrated that when lipiodol is present inside the lesion and the dimensions of the tumor do not increase, the tumor is completely necrosed [21]. It is considered that a homogenous and dense presence of lipiodol inside the lesion one month after therapy represents a sign of intratumoral necrosis [19].

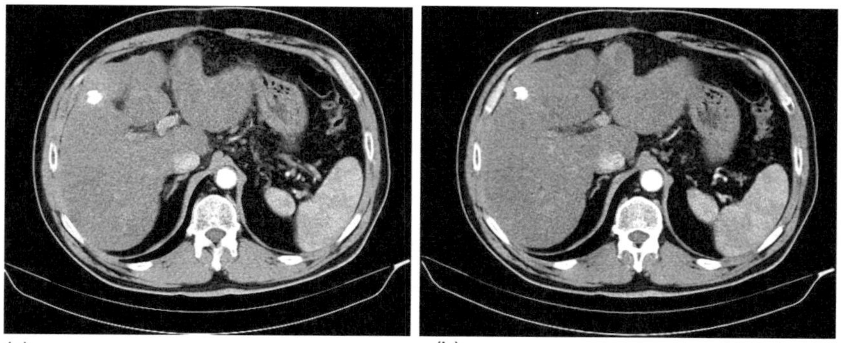

Figure 4. a. Lipiodol present inside the lesion one month after TACE. CT examination. We remark the hyperechoic, homogenous, dense aspect of the lipiodol concentrated inside the lesion. b. The same case, follow-up 3 months after treatment. We remark the persistence of lipiodol inside the lesion and a discrete decrease of tumor dimensions.

According to the recommendations of the Japanese experts, evaluation of the direct effects of treatment on the target mass (treatment effect – TE) requires the following steps [19]:

1. Tumoral necrosis and the reduction rate of the dimensions of the nodule are calculated based on the decrease in the dimensions and disappearance of nodule hypervascularization at contrast-enhanced CT examination. It is important to note that the experts accept the use of other contrast-enhanced imaging techniques such as contrast-enhanced MRI and/or contrast-enhanced ultrasound (CEUS) during follow-up as an alternative to CT scan.
2. The percentage of tumoral necrosis obtained through therapy is calculated.
3. The reduction rate of the tumor dimensions is calculated.
4. When multiple lesions are present, TE is individually determined for each lesion.

The Japanese experts classify TE as:

- TE4 when the tumor-necrotising effect is 100% or the tumor size reduction rate is 100%.
- In case of ethanol injection therapy, microwave coagulation therapy and radiofrequency ablation, TE4 is divided into TE4a (100% necrotized tumor) when the necrotized area is larger than the original nodule and TE4b when the necrotized area has the same size as the original nodule. This situation is also noted as 100% necrotized tumor, but separately classified because the risk of recurrence is higher than in TE4a cases.
- In TACE, the tendency of reduction of tumor size, without tumor enhancement on CE-CT (contrast-enhanced CT) scan, and denser uniform accumulation of lipiodol over time than just after TACE when lipiodol is used, is classified as TE4.
- TE3 defines the cases when tumor-necrotizing effect or tumor size reduction rate is between 50% and < 100%
- TE2 defines effects other than TE3 and TE1, and

- TE1 when the tumor appears enlarged by > 25% regardless of the necrotizing effect [19].

The biological marker for monitoring recurrence after any of the therapeutic procedures was, until recently, only AFP (α-fetoprotein). The specificity of AFP is high when levels are over 200 ng/ml, but with sensitivity not higher than 22% [3].

Several markers have currently been introduced in an attempt to increase the possibility of detecting primary HCC or recurrence after a curative or palliative therapeutic measure as early as possible. Of these markers, it is worth mentioning γ des-carboxi prothrombin (DPC), also known as prothrombin induced by absence of vitamin K (PIVKA). Recent clinical studies that used DPC in the detection of HCC have shown higher sensitivity and specificity compared to AFP [22].

In the global evaluation of the therapeutic effect, the Japanese experts also take into account, in the RECICL criteria, tumoral markers (α-fetoprotein, (AFP, AFP-L3) and PIVKA-II (protein induced by vitamin K absence or antagonist) or DCP (des-gamma-carboxy-prothrombin). The importance of these markers is not necessarily given by their serum levels, but more by their variations under the influence of therapy. Thus, experts consider that the lowest concentration obtained 3 months after therapy is considered to be the reference value for global evaluation of therapy, with any other increase in serum concentrations of these markers being considered an alarm signal highlighting the risk of recurrence. It is noteworthy that the *EASL-EORTC Clinical Practice Guidelines: Management of hepatocellular carcinoma* state that "accurate tumor biomarkers for early detection need to be developed" and that „Data available with tested biomarkers (i.e. AFP, AFP-L3 and DCP) show that these tests are suboptimal for routine clinical pratice (evidence 2D; recommendation 2B)", while "Use of changes in serum levels of biomarkers for the assessment of response (i.e. AFP levels) is under investigation" [3].

Another debated problem is the optimal moment for evaluating the effects of therapy. In case of evaluating local therapies (PEI, RFA or microwave coagulation therapy), effects may be assessed immediately after therapy. In case of loco-regional therapies (transcatheter arterial chemoembolization with or without lipiodol or transcatheter arterial embolization), the optimal moment for assessing therapeutic effects is considered to be after at least one month. The Japanese experts consider that global therapeutic response is at a maximum within 3 months after treatment, while in case of radiotherapy optimal evaluation is at 6 months after therapy. They recommend the use of RECIST and WHO criteria for evaluating systemic therapy and radiotherapy, including molecular targeted agents, in combination with the RECICL criteria [19].

Regarding post-therapeutic follow-up for detection of recurrence, EASL-EORTC Clinical Practice Guidelines recommend the use of a contrast-enhanced imaging examination "every 3 months during the first year, and every 6 moths thereafter to complete at least two years. Afterwards, regular ultrasound is recommended every 6 months. Assessment of time to progression is recommended with CT and/or MRI every 6-8 weeks" [3].

According to the EASL guidelines, post-therapeutic follow-up by abdominal ultrasound must be performed by qualified individuals every 3-4 months after surgical resection or after local ablative therapies (evidence 3D; recommendation 2B). [23,24]

Contrast-enhanced spiral CT scan remains the imaging technique of choice for monitoring HCC treatment, since it offers an overview of tumoral extension and is not limited by abdominal feature or liver steatosis [25]. The main problem in follow-up by CT scan is represented by the irradiation associated with repeated monitoring procedures and by renal toxicity of iodized contrast media.

MRI examination with gadolinium presents the advantage of the absence of irradiation and of increased sensitivity and specificity in detecting intratumoral vascularization, especially in small tumors [26]. The procedure is not as easliy accesible, MRI machines usually being found in tertiary centers of diagnosis and treatment. The problem of contrast-enhanced renal toxicity remains for this technique as well.

2D ultrasound examination has a low efficiency in assessing effects of therapy in HCC because it is not capable of differentiating viable tumoral tissue from post-therapeutic tumoral necrosis. It also has a limited role in detecting new lesions and in assessing the development of potential complications of local or loco-regional treatment immediately or early after the procedure. Similarly, its role in the evaluation of disease progression (portal vein thrombosis) is limited. Doppler ultrasound may sometimes identify intratumoral vascularization, but the absence of Doppler signal does not exclude the presence of viable tumoral tissue. The introduction of contrast-enhanced ultrasound (CEUS) represented an important advance, due to its capability of identifying intralesional microcirculation; CEUS has proven its efficiency in post-therapeutic follow-up as an alternative to contrast-enhanced CT or MRI. CEUS examination presents the advantage of dynamic examination, of lack of irradiation and of the possibility of repeating as often as necessary during follow-up. Second generation contrast media used in Europe are eliminated from the body through respiration, thus avoiding hepatic and renal toxicity. However, CEUS examination presents the same limits as the ultrasound method in general (operator/equipment dependent; limitations imposed by the ultrasound window, as well as post-therapeutic steatosis which appears in oncological patients and hampers profound visibility). For these reasons CEUS will not be able to totally replace the other imaging techniques.

Although in the *EASL-EORTC Clinical Practice Guidelines: Management of hepatocellular carcinoma* the roles of CEUS and angiography are considered controversial, and PET-CT "not accurate" [3], these aspects only refer to early diagnosis of HCC. The indications of CEUS are defined by the European Federation of Societies for Ultrasound in Medicine and Biology (EFSUMB) in the *"Guidelines and good clinical practice recommendations for contrast enhanced ultrasound (CEUS) – update 2008"*. The *„Update 2012"* reaches a consensus between World Federations of Ultrasound in Medicine and Biology (WFUMB) and European Federations of Ultrasound in Medicine and Biology (EFSUMB) in cooperation with representatives of other important international ultrasound societies (AFSUMB, AIUM, ASUM, FLAUS and ICUS). The Guidelines focus on its pre-, intra- and post-therapeutic role in ablative therapies for HCC, while follow-up of systemic therapies is currently regarded as an unvalidated indication. This is despite its efficiency being shown in large clinical studies [27,28]. Therefore, CEUS is recommended before treatment in addition to contrast-enhanced CT and/or MRI, but cannot exclude these examinations, which remain the examinations of choice for the diagnosis of HCC.

Another indication for CEUS is in ultrasound guiding of ablative procedures, helping to position the needle inside the tumor when it is incompletely or poorly deliniated at standard ultrasound. During the same examination CEUS allows an immediate evaluation of therapeutic response and guidance for immediate retreatment of the residual tumoral areas. The last indication is in evaluating tumoral recurrence when contrast-enhanced CT or MRI are contraindicated or inconclusive, and it is considered that CEUS can be used in protocols for post-therapeutic follow-up in association with CE-CT and CE-MRI, which remain the indications of choice for post-therapeutic follow-up, its diagnostic accuracy being equivalent to that of CE-CT or MRI [29]. Moreover, ultrasound examination 24 hours after the procedure, including CEUS, identifies not only lesion characteristics, but also potential post-interventional complications (for example bleeding).

In case of ablative procedures, CEUS examination shows a central non-enhancing area which presents a peripheral ring of homogenous hyper-enhancement determined by post-procedure inflammation. At 24 hours after the procedure, the peripheral inflammatory ring becomes thinner, the necrotic area appears larger compared to the previous examination, and the eventual residual tumor appears more evident.

The sensitivity of CT and CEUS in assessing therapeutic efficiency is however low in the first days after the procedure, especially due to post-lesional hyperemia; for this reason a contrast-enhanced imaging control is necessary one month after ablation in order to confirm the results of treatment [30]. In case of therapeutic success, further follow-up is performed according to the EASL-EORTC Clinical Practice Guidelines recommendations every 3 months by using a contrast-enhanced imaging technique (figures 5-7).

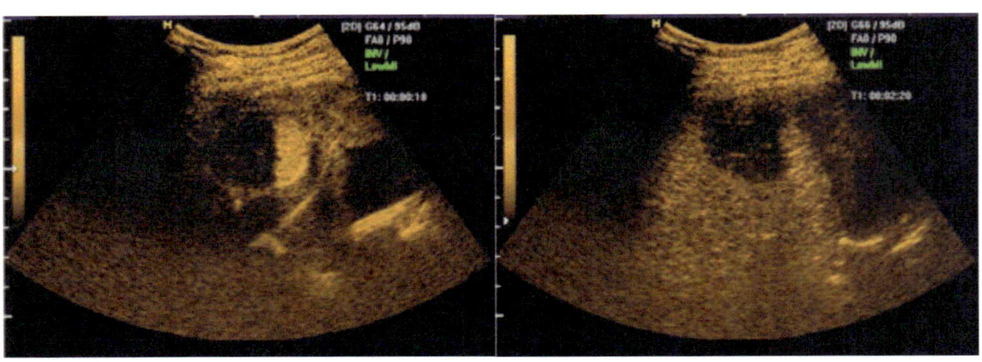

(a) (b)

Figure 5. Incomplete RFA, CEUS exam performed 3 months after therapy. Note the hyperenhancing excentric area with irregular internal contour in the arterial phase (left image) and with pronounced wash-out in the portal venous phase (right image).

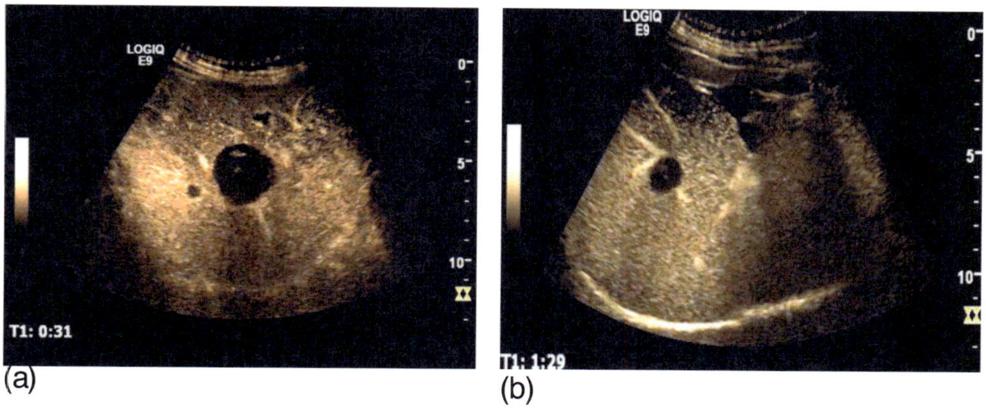

Figure 6. a. The same case, complete response after re-treatment (RFA), CEUS examination. We remark a regular internal contour of the non-enhancing area, without peripheral enhancement of the contrast media. b. The same case, a second nodule, complete response after re-treatment (RFA), CEUS examination.

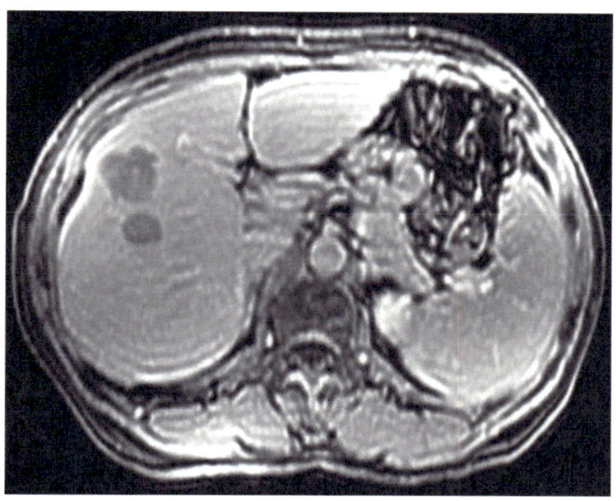

Figure 7. The same case, complete response after re-treatment (RFA) of both nodules. CE-MRI image.

A randomized study showed that recurrence at 2 years after RFA was significantly lower than after percutaneous ethanol injection. However, recurrence after RFA occurs more frequently and earlier when compared with surgical resection. Recurrence is also more frequent in case of percutaneous RFA compared to RFA through open or laparoscopic surgery, and when lesions are larger than 3 cm [31].

Transarterial chemoembolization (TACE) is based on the fact that HCC vascularization is predominantly arterial, while the remaining hepatic parenchyma has a dual nutritive vascularization (predominantly portal). For this reason TACE is effective only in lesions with hyperenhancement in the arterial phase. In cases of TACE procedures with lipiodol, immediate evaluation, as well as evaluation in the first days post-procedure, are inappropriate using CT and CEUS. Although CE-MRI is not influenced by the presence of lipiodol, it remains a costly and difficult to access method. Lipiodol may persist for months inside the lesion, and this is why assessment of therapeutic efficiency is currently done by indirectly evaluating fixation of lipiodol inside the lesion by CT without contrast media [32]. The EASL-EORTC Clinical Practice Guidelines recommend the same follow-up timing as in ablative procedures (figures 8a and b).

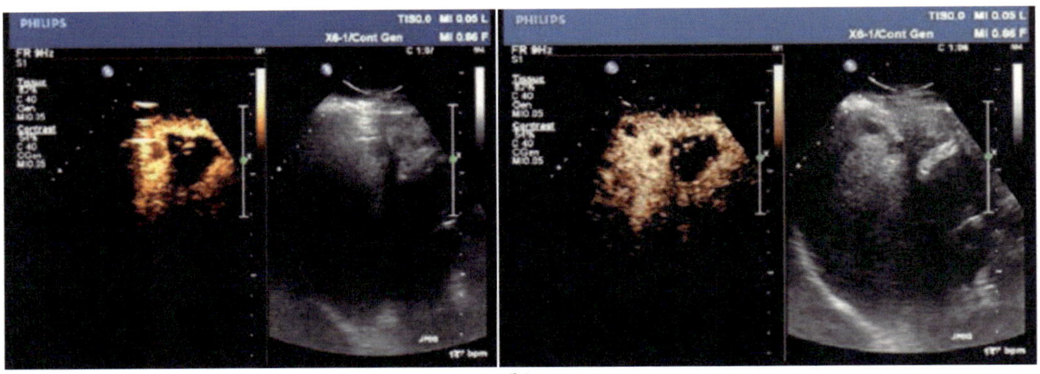

(a) (b)

Figure 8. a. Partial response after RFA and TACE. We remark the irregular, internal contour and contrast enhancement at the periphery of the lesion. b. The same case. After loco-regional therapy we also note complete necrosis of two satellite nodules of the initial tumor.

The role of ultrasound assessment is limited in the first days after the procedure and should be used only to assess for complications of the procedure. On the other hand, CEUS may play an important role during follow-up in monitoring dysplastic nodules in order to detect the moment when changes occur in arterial vascularization, facilitating therapeutic intervention as soon as possible [33].

Systemic therapies are indicated in advanced stages of hepatic tumors, when no more efficient therapeutic options remain. In addition to the recommendations for follow-up of the EASL-EORTC Clinical Practice Guidelines, CEUS has provided a significant benefit, being used in ample clinical studies to quantify intratumoral perfusion (figures 9 and 10) [34,35].

Surgical resection represents the treatment of choice for patients with a single hepatic lesion and with well conserved liver function. Recurrence rate is over 70% at 5 years and is mainly due to dissemination of the primary tumor. The appearance of new tumors near the scar of the primary tumor is considered having origin in restant tumoral cells and noted as recurrence. The most important predictors of recurrence are appearance of other tumors near the scar of the primary tumor and vascular microinvasion [36]. The EASL-EORTC Clinical Practice Guidelines recommend the same follow-up timing after resection. No increased benefit using CEUS was noted.

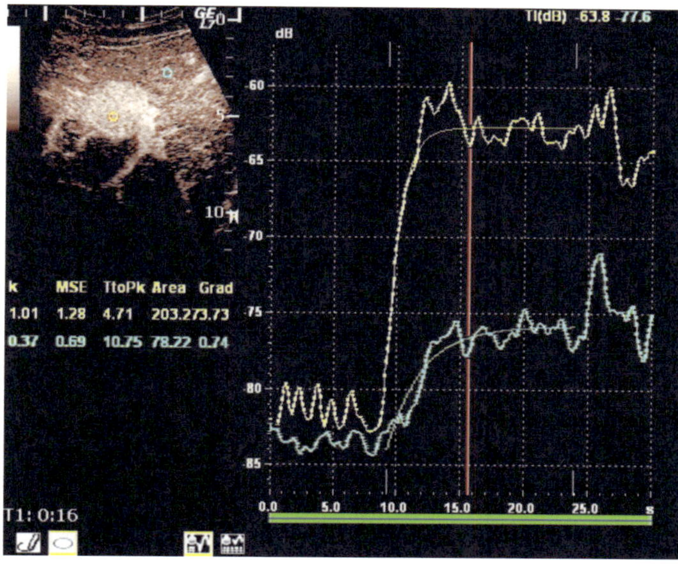

Figure 9. Quantitative analysis (time-intensity curve - TIC) of tumor vascularization before systemic therapy.

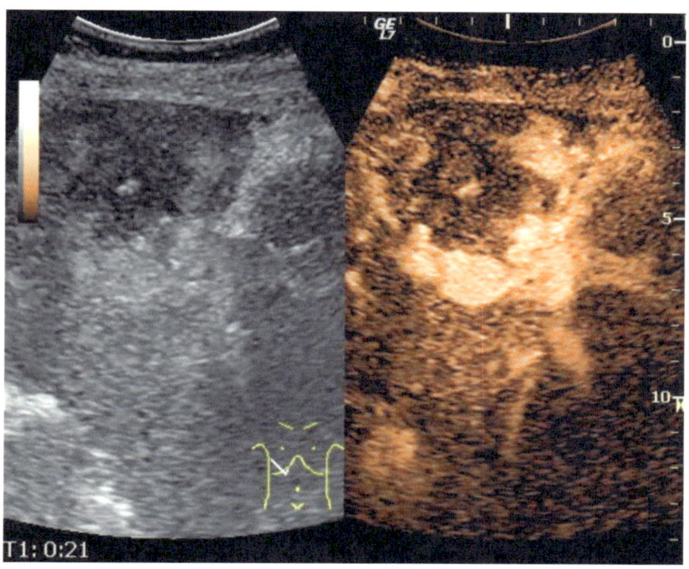

Figure 10. Therapeutic induced necrosis after Sorafenib therapy. CEUS examination, arterial phase.

3. Conclusions

Hepatocellular carcinoma is one of the most frequent malignant tumors, and its incidence is rising. HCC develops in most cases in patients with chronic liver disease, usually of viral etiology, and malignant transformation is more frequent in the cirrhotic liver. Therefore, strict follow-up of patients with liver cirrhosis is recommended in order to diagnose HCC as early as possible.

Carcinogenesis is a complex, multistep and multicentric process. Changes in the intratumoral vascularization are specific to HCC and allow for its imaging-based diagnosis. Several therapeutic options are available, depending on the stage of the tumor. Thus, surgical resection or local therapies are recommended in early stages, while loco-regional and systemic therapies or radiotherapy are indicated for intermediate and advanced stages.

A very important role is played by post-therapeutic follow-up, which includes complex criteria for assessing both the direct effect of therapy on the tumoral nodule (tumoral necrosis induced by treatment and variations of tumor dimensions) as well as global therapeutic response (appearance of complications of HCC or of liver cirrhosis and development of new tumoral nodules) – the mRECIST and RECICL criteria.

The imaging techniques of choice for the early diagnosis of recurrences are represented by contrast-enhanced CT and contrast-enhanced MRI. CEUS represents a viable alternative for post-therapeutic follow-up, because it has a diagnostic accuracy similar to that of the other two techniques and has the advantages of lack of irradiation and lack of hepatic and renal toxicity; however CEUS cannot replace the two other techniques. CEUS is recommended to be used in post-therapeutic follow-up together with CE-CT and CE-MRI.

Although the role of serum tumoral markers in the diagnosis of HCC is considered to be "suboptimal" while their variations during evolution are "under investigation", they are still used in current clinical practice, especially for post-therapeutic follow-up.

Author details

Simona Ioaniţescu[1], L. Micu[1], Mariana Mihăilă[1] and R. Badea[2]

1 Center of Internal Medicine, Fundeni Clinical Institute, Bucharest, Romania

2 Ultrasound Dept., Institute of Gastroenterology and Hepatology, Univ. of Medicine & Pharmacy "Iuliu Haţieganu"Cluj-Napoca, Romania

References

[1] Ferlay J, Bray F, Pisani P, Parkin DM. GLOBOCAN 2000: cancer incidence, mortality and prevalence worldwide, version 1.0. International Agency for Research on Cancer CancerBase no. 5. Lyon, France: IARC Press, 2001.

[2] Surveillance, Epidemiology, and End Results (SEER) Program. SEER*Stat database: incidence — SEER 9 Regs research data, Nov 2009 Sub (1973-2007). Bethesda, MD: National Cancer Institute, April 2010.

[3] European Association for the Study of the Liver and European Organisation for Research and Treatment of Cancer. EASL-EORTC Clinical Practice Guidelines: management of hepatocellular carcinoma," Journal of Hepatology, vol 56, pp. 908-943, 2012.

[4] Takayama T, Makuuchi M, Hirohashi S, Sakamoto M, Yamamoto J, Shimada K, et al. Early hepatocellular carcinoma as an entity with a high rate of surgical cure. Hepatology 1998;28:1241–1246.

[5] Roayaie S, Blume IN, Thung SN, Guido M, Fiel MI, Hiotis S, et al. A system of classifying microvascular invasion to predict outcome after resection in patients with hepatocellular carcinoma. Gastroenterology 2009;137:850–855.

[6] Roayaie S, Llovet JM, Obeidat K, Labow D, Sposito C, Pellegrinelli A, et al. Hepatic resection for hepatocellular carcinoma < 2 cm in diameter. Hepatology, in press.

[7] Livraghi T, Meloi F, Di Stasi M, Rolle E, Solbiati L, Tinelli C, et al. Sustained complete response and complications rates after radiofrequency ablation of very early hepatocellular carcinoma in cirrhosis: is resection still the treatment of choice? Hepatology 2008;47:82–89.

[8] Shiratoli Y, Shiina S, Imamura M, et al: Characteristic difference of hepatocellular carcinoma between hepatitis B- and C-viral infection in Japan. Hepatology 1995;22:1027–1033.

[9] Llovet JM, Burroughs A, Bruix J. Hepatocellular carcinoma. Lancet 2003;362:1907–1917.

[10] Fattovich G, Stroffolini T, Zagni I, Donato F. Hepatocellular carcinoma in cirrhosis: incidence and risk factors. Gastroenterology 2004; 127: S35-S50

[11] Andreana L, Isgrò G, Pleguezuelo M, Germani G, Burroughs A. Surveillance and diagnosis of hepatocellular carcinoma in patients with cirrhosis. World J Hepatol 2009 October 31; 1(1): 48-61

[12] Burrel M, Llovet JM, Ayuso C, Iglesias C, Sala M, Miquel R, Caralt T, Ayuso JR, Sole M, Sanchez M, Bru C, Bruix J. MRI angiography is superior to helical CT for detection of HCC prior to liver transplantation: an explant correlation. Hepatology 2003;38:1034-1042

[13] Caturelli E, Bartolucci F, Biasini E, Vigliotti ML, Andriulli A, Siena DA, Attino V, Bisceglia M. Diagnosis of liver nodules observed in chronic liver disease patients during ultrasound screening for early detection of hepatocellular carcinoma. Am J Gastroenterol 2002; 97: 397-405

[14] Matsui O. Imaging of multistep human hepatocarcinogenesis by CT during intra-arterial contrast injection. Intervirology 2004;47:271-276.

[15] Lencioni R, Piscaglia F, Bolondi L. Contrast-enhanced ultrasound in the diagnosis of hepatocellular carcinoma. Journal of Hepatology (2008);48:848–857

[16] Lencioni R, Llovet J.M. Modified RECIST (mRECIST) Assessment for Hepatocellular Carcinoma. Semin Liver Dis 2010;30:52-60

[17] Eisenhauer E.A, Therasse P, Bogaerts J, Schwartz L.H, Sargent D, Ford R, Dancey J, Arbuck S, Gwyther S, Mooney M, Rubinstein L, Shankar L, Dodd L, Kaplan R, Lacombe D, Verweij J. New response evaluation criteria in solid tumours: Revised RECIST guideline (version 1.1). EJC (2009); 45:228 –247. doi:10.1016/j.ejca.2008.10.026

[18] D'Amico G, Garcia-Tsao G, Pagliaro L. Natural history and prognostic indicators of survival in cirrhosis: a systematic review of 118 studies. J Hepatol 2006;44(1):217–231

[19] Kudo M, Kubo S, Takayasu K, Sakamoto M, Tanaka M, Ikai I, Furuse J, Nakamura K, Makuuchi M. Response evaluation criteria in cancer of the liver (RECICL) proposed by the Liver Cancer Study Group of Japan (2009 Revised Version). Hepatology Research 2010;40:686-692 DOI: 10.1111/j.1872-034x.2010.00674.x

[20] Sparchez Z; Radu P; Zaharia T; Kacso G; Grigorescu I; Botis G; Badea R. Usefulness of contrast enhanced ultrasound guidance in percutaneous biopsies of liver tumors. JGLD 2011;20(2):191 - 196.

[21] Takayasu K, Arii S, Matsuo N et al. Comparison of CT findings with resected specimens after chemoembolization with iodized oil for hepatocellular carcinoma. Am J Roentgenol 2000; 175: 699–704.

[22] Carr B.I, Wang Z, Wei G. Differential effects of vitamin K1 on AFP and DPC leveles in patients with unresecable HCC and HCC cell lines. Digestive Disease and Sciences 2011;56(6):1876-1883.

[23] Bruix J, Sherman M, Llovet JM, Beaugrand M, Lencioni R, Burroughs AK, et al. EASL Panel of Experts on HCC. Clinical management of hepatocellular carcinoma. Conclusions of the Barcelona-2000 EASL conference. European Association for the Study of the Liver. J Hepatol 2001;35:421–430.

[24] National Cancer Institute. PDQ_ levels of evidence for adult and pediatric cancer treatment studies. Bethesda, MD: National Cancer Institute. Date last modified 26/August/2010. <http://cancer.gov/cancertopics/pdq/levelsevidence- adult-treatment/healthprofessional/>; 2011 [accessed 01.03.11].

[25] Bartolozzi C, Cioni D, Donati F, Granai G, Lencioni R. Imaging evaluation of tumor response. In: Bartolozzi C, Lencioni R, editors. Liver malignancies. Diagnostic and interventional radiology, 1st ed. Berlin: Springer-Verlag, 1999. pp. 467–487.

[26] Dromain C, de Baere T, Elias D, et al. Hepatic tumors treated with percutaneous radiofrequency ablation: CT and MR imaging follow up. Radiology 2002; 223: 255-262.

[27] Claudon, M, Cosgrove, D, Albrecht, T, Bolondi, L, Bosio, M, Calliada, F, Correas, J-M, Darge, K, Dietrich, C, D'Onofrio, M, Evans, D. H, Filice, C, Greiner, L, Jäger, K, de Jong, N, Leen, E, Lencioni, R, Lindsell, D, Martegani, A, Meairs, S, Nolsøe, C, Piscaglia, F, Ricci, P, Seidel, G, Skjoldbye, B, Solbiati, L, Thorelius, L, Tranquart, F, We-

skott, H-P, Whittingham, T. Guidelines and Good Clinical Practice Recommendations for Contrast Enhanced Ultrasound (CEUS) - update 2008. Ultraschall Med (2008). , 29, 28-44.

[28] Claudon M, Dietrich CF., Choi BI, Cosgrove DO,Kudo M, Nolsøe CP, Piscaglia F, Wilson SR, Barr RG, Chammas MC, Chaubal NG, Chen M-H, Clevert DA, Correas JM, Ding H, Forsberg F, Fowlkes JB, RN Gibson, Goldberg BB, Lassau N, Leen E. L. S, Mattrey R. F, Moriyasu F, Solbiati L, Weskott H-P, Xu H-X. Guidelines and Good Clinical Practice Recommendations for Contrast Enhanced Ultrasound (CEUS) in the Liver – Update 2012. A WFUMB-EFSUMB initiative in cooperation with representatives of AFSUMB, AIUM, ASUM, FLAUS and ICUS. Ultraschall in Med 2012; DOI: 10.1055/s-0032-1325499.

[29] Frieser M, et al. Efficacy of Contrast-Enhanced US versus CT or MRI for the Therapeutic Control of Percutaneous Radiofrequency Ablation in the Case of Hepatic Malignancies. Ultraschall in Med. Published online 2011. ISSN: 0172-4614.

[30] Nicolau C, Vilana R, Bianchi L, Brú C. Early-stage hepatocellular carcinoma: the high accuracy of real-time contrast-enhanced ultrasonography in the assessment of response to percutaneous treatment. Eur Radiol 2007; 17(Suppl 6): F80-88.

[31] Khan KN, Yattsuhashi H, Yamasaki K, Inouc O, Koga M, et al. Prospective analysis of risk factors for early intrahepatic recurrence of hepatocellular carcinoma following ethanol injection. J Hepatol. 2000; 32: 269-278.

[32] Maruyama H, Yoshikawa M, Yokosuka O. Current role of ultrasound for the management of hepatocellular carcinoma. World J Gastroenterol 2008; 14: 1710-1719

[33] Badea R, Ioanitescu S. Ultrasound Imaging of Liver Tumors – Current Clinical Applications. In: "Liver Tumors". Alexander Julianov (ed.). InTech, Rijeca, Croatia, 2012, pp. 75 – 102. http://www.intechopen.com/books/liver-tumors/ultrasound-imaging-of-liver-tumors-current-clinical-applications (accessed 5.09.2012)

[34] Yoshida K, Hirokawa T, Moriyasu F, Liu L, Liu G-J, Yamada M, Imai Y. Arterial-phase contrast-enhanced ultrasonography for evaluating anti-angiogenesis treatment: A pilot study. World J Gastroenterol 2011 February 28; 17(8): 1045-1050. doi: 10.3748/wjg.v17.i8.1045.

[35] Lassau N, Chami L, Chebil M, Benatsou B, Bidault S, Girard E, Abboud G, Roche A. Dynamic Contrast-Enhanced Ultrasonography (DCE-US) and Anti-angiogenic Treatments. Discov Med 11(56):18-24, January 2011.

[36] Bruix J, Sherman M. Management of hepatocellular carcinoma. Hepatology 2005;42: 1208–1236.

Chapter 7

Liver Metastases — Surgical Treatment

Alejandro Serrablo, Luis Tejedor and
Jose-Manuel Ramia

Additional information is available at the end of the chapter

http://dx.doi.org/10.5772/55898

1. Introduction

Liver metastases are now detected at earlier stages because of the improvement in imaging techniques and the closer follow-up of cancer patients. The right lobe is metastasized to more frequently than the left, mainly due to the preference of tumour emboli circulating through the right portal vein as a feature of the portal stream. Liver metastases may also arise from draining lymphnodes through venolymphatics communications or the thoracic duct [1]. Lymphatic metastases may arise from these portal blood born liver metastases, usually pointing to a very poor prognosis.

All patients with colorectal liver metastases (CLM) are classified as having stage IV disease in the TNM classification of liver tumours given by the International Union Against Cancer (UICC) and the American Joint Committee on Cancer (AJCC), but they form a very heterogeneous group (synchronous and metachronous metastases, node-positive and node-negative disease, unilobar and bilobar lesions, and extrahepatic or no extrahepatic disease) and their long-term outcomes may vary widely. Several clinical scores [2-6], based on retrospective data, have been developed to predict more accurately the prognosis of these patients and thus to stratify their management, but their validation is still limited.

2. Colorectal liver metastases

The liver is the most frequent and often unique site of metastasis in patients with colorectal cancer, both at the time of diagnosis (20–25% of cases) or after an apparently radical surgery on the primary tumour (40% of cases) [7]. Less than one third of patients with CLM have disease limited to one lobe and in only 10% of cases is metastasis solitary.

CLM are usually asymptomatic but patients may develop abdominal discomfort, weight loss, general malaise and hepatomegaly with advanced disease. Jaundice, ascites and occasionally portal hypertension are late signs. Pain and fever related to necrosis and infarction of a metastasis are usually transient symptoms.

CLM are often harder to palpate than the normal liver, extend by concentric growth and may spread to other structures by penetrating the usually rigid Glisson´s capsule.

The natural history of metastatic colorectal cancer is variable. Median survival without treatment is less than eight months from presentation but the prognosis is better for those patients with isolated CLM. Survival of patients with untreated CLM at five years is unusual.

2.1. Diagnosis

Diagnosis of CLM is mainly based in imaging studies, with history, physical examination and serum levels of alkaline phosphatase, aspartate aminotrasaminase, glutamyl transferase and carcinoembryonic antigen playing a minor role. Accurate detection of CLM has important prognostic implications, since untreated liver metastases have a poor prognosis (5-year survival rate of 0-3%) while the resection with curative intent offers a much better one (5-year survival rate from 35% to 58%) [8]. The imaging of these lesions, needed for a careful pre-operative selection of patients, should assess their number, size and segmental location, their differential diagnosis with benign lesions, possible hilar lymph node involvement (although the pre-operative diagnosis is difficult), the evaluation of vascular invasion, the liver volume (insufficient residual volume of liver parenchyma is a contraindication to surgery), and the presence of extrahepatic disease (although peritoneal carcinomatosis is very difficult to detect.

The specificity of imaging studies detecting CLM is higher than 85%, and the sensitivity for detection of liver metastases is progressively increasing from transabdominal ultrasound (US) to multi-detector computed tomography (CT), magnetic resonance imaging (MRI) and fluorodeoxyglucose-enhanced positron emission tomography (FDG PET) [9]. FDG PET and CT can be combined to provide fused images, achieving high spatial resolution and functional information in the same images (FDG PET/CT).

Biopsy of suspected CLM is not usually done in patients with potentially resectable disease because imaging studies are generally accurate enough and percutaneous biopsy may be asociated with extrahepatic dissemination.

CT scan remains the dominant imaging modality both for detection of CLM and preoperative planning as well as for treatment monitoring and post-treatment surveillance. CT combined with FDG PET/CT may avoid additional studies and may improve patient management [32-34]. Contrast-enhanced MRI should be reserved for problem solving. Because MRI sensitivity in detecting extrahepatic disease in the peritoneum and chest is low, it is not a desirable primary imaging modality.

2.1.1. Ultrasonography

US is a rapid and non-invasive method for screening patients with suspected liver metastases. While it is highly efficient in distinguishing patients with diffuse hepatic metastases, it is more operator dependent than other imaging studies and its sensitivity (50-70%) and specificity are surpassed by other imaging methods.

Contrast-enhanced US (CEUS) improves the sensitivity compared to conventional B-mode sonography by using microbubbles of gas that flood the blood pool after intravenous injection. Metastases show characteristic images in arterial, portal and delayed phases, thereby increasing CEUS sensitivity and specificity in staging liver metastases and approaching those of CT and MRI [8]. As CEUS improves the detection of metastases smaller than 1 cm and of those lesions that are isoechoic with respect to adjacent liver parenchyma, it improves the performance of US in around 13.7% of the cases [10]. CEUS can be suboptimal in visualizing certain parts of the liver, especially in obese patients and/or in cases of steatosis and may find difficult to differentiate hypervascular metastases from haemangiomas and metastases from small cysts [11]. For these reasons, US should not be the imaging method of choice in the assessment of CLM.

2.1.2. Computed tomography

CT sensitivity and specificity are high (70–85% and 90% respectively) especially for lesions bigger than 1.5–2 cm. Although sensitivity is lower for small subglissonian metastases, multislice CT enables detection of lesions of 0.5 cm in size (thicknesses of 2 or 4 mm are the most effective for detection of focal liver lesions, with an identical detection rate of 96% for both) [12]. Fast data acquisition allows bi-phasic contrast-enhanced scan during the arterial-dominant and the portal perfusion phases after bolus contrast administration, prior to the equilibrium phase (hepatic venous or interstitial). This part of the study should be considered as standard for the optimised view of the complex vascularization of the liver and potential hepatic lesions.

CT can be used for evaluating the liver lesion, liver parenchyma and hepatic vessels in the same sitting, since its software grants 3-D data sets, which improves multiplanar imaging, demonstrates the vascular anatomy and characterizes the lesions well. This feature, together with improvements in bolus-tracking, facilitates CT-angiography of the liver and mesenteric vessels, which can be invaluable in patients undergoing hepatic resection or transarterial chemo or radio-embolisation. The CT portal venogram is useful in evaluation of the portal system. Quantitative perfusion studies can also be done.

CT software is also able to highlight different liver segments, assess liver volume and to create vascular maps for arterial and portal inflow and hepatic venous drainage, which are necessary in evaluating the feasibility of major hepatectomies. A simulation of surgical resection can be performed. This information can be shown visually using coloured maps or three-dimensional movies [13], which are tools increasingly used because they ease surgical dissection but still requiring validation.

The utility of CT as a pre-operative tool to evaluate CLM is inversely proportional to the time elapsed between imaging and surgery, which may explain the conflicting reports on the accuracy of CT [14].

2.1.3. *Magnetic resonance imaging*

Although CT is usually preferred because of its availability and its good surveillance of the extrahepatic abdominal organs and tissues, MRI has an advantage in the characterization of focal lesions. It is also used for patients who cannot receive intravenous iodinated contrast material or there is concerns about the risk of radiation from repeated exposure to CT. MRI sensitivity and specificity (85-90% and up to 95% respectively) are higher than those of CT, but this comparison needs to be reassessed periodically, owing to the rapid evolution of both technologies.

The extracellular agent gadolinium-chelate complex is the most commonly used contrast media in dynamic MRI. The current standard MRI liver protocol includes a T2-weighted sequence, a T1-weighted sequence and a three-phase technique after administration of gadolinium. Detection of CLM is maximized during the portal venous phase, like in CT scan. Organ-specific contrast agents with hepatocyte specificity (mangafodipir trisodium [MnDPDP], gadobenate dimeglumine [Gd-BOPTA]) or reticuloendothelial system specificity (superparamagnetic iron oxide [SPIO] particles, captured by Kupffer cells) increase the sensitivity and specificity [15,16], but data about their benefits are controversial and they are generally expensive and not widely available.

Diffusion-weighted MR imaging (DWI) depict differences in molecular diffusion caused by the random motion of molecules without the need for a contrast agent [8] and can obtain quantitative indices, helpful in the assessment of disease response to novel therapeutics (including antivascular and anti-angiogenic therapy) [17]. It can be a simple and sensitive method for screening focal hepatic lesions and very useful for differential diagnosis [18].

2.1.4. *Positron emission tomography*

FDG PET sensitivity and specificity are high for CLM (92–100% and 85–100% respectively). However, false negative and false positive findings in FDG PET for CLM are not negligible [19] and its positive predictive value (PPV) is not high. Thus, some teams recommend histological confirmation when the findings suggests non-resectability [20]. Some studies have demonstrated high diagnostic values of FDG PET in the evaluation of liver metastases [21-23] confirming its superior sensitivity on a per patient basis, but not on a per lesion basis. Nevertheless, its role is not yet clear owing to the small number of studies [24].

In the context of CLM, FDG PET/CT may avoid unnecessary surgery when it detects extrahepatic foci of disease that are not depicted or characterized as malignant by other imaging methods [25]. When these patients have a FDG PET prior to surgery, there is a lower probability of non-therapeutic laparotomy [26] and an improved survival [27], reflecting better patient selection. As a drawback, this technology is not suitable for liver resection planning.

2.1.5. *Intraoperative ultrasonography*

The best standard of reference when comparing diagnostic studies is laparotomy with bimanual palpation and intraoperative ultrasonography (IOUS). This method finds additional lesions in 33% of patients with preoperative diagnosed CLM and new lesions in 5% of patients without known CLM [1].

IOUS has higher sensitivity (98%) than transabdominal US, CT and MRI (its specificity is 95%), allows the detection of lesions 0.5 cm in size and defines the relationship between lesion, vessels and biliary structures. It is generally considered the gold standard for detecting liver lesions and is regarded as a routine investigation, since it modifies the planned surgical strategy in 18-30% of the patients. In addition, Doppler and spectral Doppler facilitate the technique of surgical resection.

Laparoscopy allows an assessment of the peritoneal spread, liver surface, extrahepatic disease and vessel invasion. Its combination with laparoscopic ultrasound (LIOUS) modifies the initial surgical plan in 20–30% of the cases [12].

Contrast enhanced IOUS (CEIOUS) shows some benefit over pre-operative imaging and IOUS since it improves the ability to characterize already detected lesions and facilitate the detection of new ones [28-31].

2.2. Surgical treatment

2.2.1. Resectable CLM

Hepatic resection offers the only chance of long-term survival for patients with CLM, the first large series concluding that there was a benefit for surgery in selected patients with CLM being reported in 1978 [35]. The 5-year survival rate for these patients has increased from about 30% two decades ago to nearly 60% nowadays, with a 10-year overall survival of 20–25% for radically resected patients [36].

Criteria for resectability

The resectability rate has improved thanks to pre-operative imaging techniques, patient selection, surgical techniques, postoperative care and new cytotoxic and biologic agents for preoperative and post-operative treatment. Thereby, the criteria for resectability of these cases have changed dramatically. The number of lesions (1 to 3 unilobar metastases), the size of the lesion (less than 5 cm), the interval of time (preferably presenting at least 12 months after resection of the primary tumour), the minimum margin of 1 cm in width and the absence of hilar adenopathy or extrahepatic disease, are no longer considered as determinant factors when considering resectability.

The number of metastases is not a risk factor for long-term survival providing that a R0 resection (complete resection with no microscopic residual tumour) has been achieved [37]. Some studies have shown that the degree of response to chemotherapy is a stronger predictor factor for longterm survival than the number of metastasis. Although reports have been conflicting, evidence shows that size is not a resectability factor, but a factor related to tumour aggressiveness. Likewise, the width of the surgical margin has no effect on survival whenever the margin is microscopically negative [38-40], though resection planning should aim for an optimum margin, i.e. greater than one centimeter in width. Extrahepatic disease was considered a contraindication to liver resection until few years ago. Five-year survival rates of 12% to 37% after hepatic resection in selected patients, independent of the location of the extrahepatic disease (lung, primary colorectal recurrence, retroperitoneal or hepatic pedicle lymph nodes, peritoneal carcinomatosis, miscellaneous) have been reported [41-45]. In most of the patients, peritoneal disease is regarded as a contraindication to hepatic resection, but can be considered in cases of stable or chemo-responsive disease when an R0 resection is achievable. These patients should be classified as having borderline resectability [46]. Positive hilar lymph nodes have been associated with a poor survival and are also generally considered as a contraindication to liver resection of CLM. Again, however, some studies have shown lengthy survival in some patients, particularly if involved nodes are limited to the hepatoduodenal-retropancreatic area [47,48], although this nodes are not routinely removed.

In short, only two criteria for resectability are universally meaningful: (1) It must be possible to remove all disease with a negative margin; (2) There must be adequate remaining hepatic reserve. The only traditional prognostic indicator of recurrence that precludes long-term survival is a positive resection margin [34].

Accordingly, CLM are considered as resectable when they can be completely resected, two adjacent liver segments can be spared while sustaining an adequate vascular inflow and outflow and biliary drainage, and the volume of the future liver remnant (FLR) is adequate (at least 20% of the total estimated volume for liver with normal parenchyma, 30–60% for liver with chemotherapy, steatosis or hepatitis, 40–70% for liver with cirrhosis) [46]. To assess resectability clinically it is useful to estimate FLR to body weight ratio, which should be greater than 0.5. However, there is no universaly adopted guideline for "resectability" of primary or metastatic liver cancer and often the experience of the individual surgeon plays an essential role.

Chemotherapy

Optimal regimens and timing of chemotherapies when liver resection is possible are unclear. The efficacy of the peri-operative chemotherapy on survival for resectable liver metastases has not been justified. Some authors suggest that treatment of resectable CLM, in the absence of high-risk features, should begin with surgery and then consider adjuvant chemotherapy [2]. There is no evidence to support neoadjuvant chemotherapy in patients with resectable disease [49]. Moreover, since around 7% of tumours will progress while on chemotherapy, this approach may compromise a few patient's chance of cure if routinely used. If high-risk features are present, most physicians prefer a short course of systemic pre-operative chemotherapy. Patients with a perforated tumour or a considerable lymphatic burden are considered candidates for neoadjuvant chemotherapy before liver surgery. The EORTC 40983 study evaluated peri-operative chemotherapy vs. surgery alone in resectable hepatic metastases and did not demonstrate a clear advantage of preoperative chemotherapy in patients with resectable CLM. Neither could this study determine if neoadjuvant, adjuvant or peri-operative chemotherapy was superior. In this trial, the postoperative complication rate was significantly increased in those patients who received perioperative chemotherapy versus surgery alone. Some of these complications were biliary fistula, hepatic failure, intra-abdominal infection, and the need for re-operation. Supporters of peri-operative treatment point out that surgery is facilitated and that the treatment provides information on tumour biology. The same study demonstrated that no patient progressed to an unresectable condition, that short cycles of treatment provided minimal liver toxicity and that survival improved in the chemotherapy sub-group [50]. Livers affected by chemotherapy are usually more rigid, more difficult to manage and tend to bleed more easily at surgery. Moreover, questions about the management of "ghost lesions" after complete response, that cannot be detected with IOUS, remain unanswered.

When resection is considered appropriate, it is imperative to have a high quality abdominopelvic CT (or MRI) within a month of the date of surgery. A chest CT should be done at that time.

Resection

Detailed knowledge of liver anatomy, inflow and outflow control, low central venous pressure, IOUS, ultrasonic dissection, argon beam coagulation, etc. contribute to reduce blood loss during the resection of CLM. Intraoperative bleeding is the main cause of postoperative morbidity and mortality since blood transfusion is associated to a decreased long-term survival, an increased perioperative mortality, a higher complication rate, a longer hospital stay, and an increased risk of infectious complications [51].

Hepatic segmentectomy, based on Couinaud segments, is preferable for localize lesions; a non-segmental resection may be technically more difficult and compromise the vascularity of adjacent residual liver. Nevertheless, IOUS must be used before attempting a wedge resection of an apparently superficial nodule. For larger or multiple CLM, standard anatomical resections must be employed. Additionally, the Brisbane 2000 Terminology of Liver Anatomy and Resections is recommended to avoid confusion in the terms used when describing surgical techniques [52].

The inability to obtain a free surgical margin during liver resection for CLM should not be a contraindication to surgery, provided complete macroscopic removal of all metastatic lesions is achieved (positive margins or R1 resection), since survival is similar to that of R0 resection, despite a higher recurrence rate (5-year and 10-year overall survival rates are 61% and 43% in R0 vs. 57% and 37% in the R1) [53].

Laparoscopic liver resection are now more frequently performed since the first one reported in 1992 [54]. It shows advantages in the short term over open surgery but there are still no data to indicate the impact of this procedure on long term outcome.

Mortality is less than 5% and morbidity is around 30%, given the wide variations in surgical aggressiveness. Postoperative hepatic failure can be a lethal complication. This depends on the volume and the function of the residual liver. In general, the larger the hepatic resection the greater the probability of postoperative complications. Other complications that may contribute to or be related to postoperative liver failure include haemorrhage, bile leak, intra-abdominal sepsis, and cardiopulmonary dysfunction.

In regard to surgery of synchronous and metachronous CLM, simultaneous colon and liver resection has been shown to be safe and efficient, since prognosis is not dependent on the time of resection of CLM.

2.2.2. Initially non-resectable CLM

Some techniques may be used when CLM are not at first resectable because of an insufficient FLR. Strategies to increase the volume of the hepatic remnant include conversion chemotherapy, portal vein occlusion, staged liver resection and combination of these procedures. Also, ablative techniques may be considered alone or in conjunction with resection.

Chemotherapy

Chemotherapy leads to improved survival in patients with unresectable CLM. In these cases, upfront chemotherapy in asymptomatic patients compared with resection of the primary tumour does not seem to affect survival significantly. However, without liver resection 60% of the patients are alive after 2 years so that resection of the primary lesion for palliative reasons and local control is recommended in rectal cancer [55].

The goal of conversion chemotherapy is downsizing the tumour for re-considering its resection. New chemotherapeutic regimens combining 5-FU, folinic acid and oxaliplatin (FOLFOX) and/or irinotecan (FOLFIRI) have improved response rates (approximately 50%), enabling 10-30% of the patients with initially unresectable disease to be operated [56]. Combined with biologic agents that target angiogenesis (bevacizumab) and the epidermal growth factor receptor (EGFR) in K-ras wildtype tumours (cetuximab), response rates of up to 70% are achieved [34]. A new re-evaluation for resection should be done after 2 or 3 months of pre-operative chemotherapy and every 2 months thereafter. Hepatic arterial infusion (HAI) of chemotherapy may be added to systemic therapy, obtaining a higher concentration of drugs in the liver with less systemic toxicity. Although response rates are higher than systemic chemotherapy, survival does not change so far. Furthermore, its complication rates are so high (57%) that it is discarded as a first option.

Chemotherapy should be stopped when the CLM have been downsized to the point where hepatic resection is possible in order to reduce liver toxicity and to avoid a complete clinical response. A complete response on CT scan does not mean cure since in over 80% of the cases there are viable cancer cells in the initial site of the metastasis [57]. These ghost lesions have to be removed or ablated, considering the FLR [58-60].

Tumour progression is associated with a poor outcome, even after potentially curative hepatectomy. Therefore, tumour control before surgery is crucial to offer a chance of prolonged remission in patients with multiple metastases [56]. Only 50% of tumours can be expected to show a partial response to chemotherapy. Patients deemed to be resectable during systemic treatment should be considered as surgical candidates regardless of the associated adverse predictive factors.

Peri-operative complications, including hepatobiliary complications, are more frequent with lengthy pre-operative chemotherapy, probably related to the prolonged and sequential use of multiple regimens [61]. Adjuvant treatment, usually FOLFOX, may be used following surgery, but HAI combined with systemic chemotherapy is also an option. Trials examining the role of adjuvant chemotherapy are difficult to conduct because of the rapidly changing chemotherapy regimens and drugs [62]. Since post-operative morbidity affects long-term survival [63], length of chemotherapy treatment must be taken into account. In recent years more and more patients with stable long-term disease (more than 20 months) are considered for surgical treatment.

Portal vein occlusion

When the FLR is insufficient portal vein occlusion should be considered. In 1990 Makuuchi presented the portal vein embolization (PVE) of the right portal branch to induce hypertrophy of the left side of the liver, enabling a safer removal of large or multiple tumours, mostly located in the right hemiliver and segment IV [64]. The rationale behind this approach is to induce atrophy of the tumour-bearing lobe with subsequent hypertrophy in the contralateral lobe by diverting the portal venous flow into the liver section that is expected to remain. In general, two methods of portal vein occlusion can be employed: PVE or surgical portal vein ligation (PVL). Neither technique has clear advantage.

Portal occlusion increases the FLR between 10% to 46% within 2 to 8 weeks and enables a R0-resection in 70% to 100% of selected cases. However, some patients show tumour progression after PVE, but it is not clear whether this is just a matter of time (from portal vein occlusion to operation) or is due to growth stimuli to the tumour by the induced liver regeneration. Portal vein occlusion also constitutes a dynamic pre-operative test on the capacity of the liver to respond to the surgical aggression: If a hypertrophy greater than 5% is achieved, there is a low risk of a severe post-operative liver insufficiency [65].

The concomitant administration of chemotherapy may decrease both the tumour load and the post-operative recurrences. Chemotherapy does not seem to affect the hypertrophy induced by PVE. A few studies using bevazucimab recommend a 6 week waiting period before surgery, although its influence on the hypertrophy is unclear.

Percutaneous PVE is usually well tolerated with minimum side effects such as fever, nausea, and transient abnormality of liver function test, and with a complication rate below 5% [66]. Major liver surgery after PVE has a complication rate of 1% for the PVE itself and a complication rate of 8.8% for the subsequent resection [67]. It increases the feasibility of liver resection by 19%. The actuarial survival rate after surgery is 40% at 5 years, similar to that of patients resected without PVE [68].

Two-stage hepatectomy

It is the combination of two sequential and planned liver resections when it is impossible to resect all liver metastases in a single procedure, while preserving at least 30% of functional liver volume to avoid post-operative liver failure. The first surgery attempts to resect the majority of CLM and to get hypertrophy of the remnant liver. The technique should be planned well in advance to achieve complete removal, admitting that around 30% of patients will not be rescued on the second hepatectomy.

Usually, on the first hepatectomy the FLR is cleared out of tumours with non-anatomic resections and/or radiofrequency ablation or at most a single segment resection [69]. This first stage can also be performed together with laparoscopic or open colorectal resection. After a period of recovery of 4 to 6 weeks and subsequent hypertrophy of the tumour-free lobe, tumour removal is completed by resection of the larger tumour mass in the contralateral liver lobe.

The majority of patients in whom this approach failed, did so because they had developed disease progression in the meantime.

As another option, two to four weeks after the first stage PVE may be performed [70]. The second surgery can be done on the fourth or fifth week after PVE, when a CT confirms that an adequate hypertrophy of the non-embolized hemi-liver is achieved. Alternatively, portal vein occlusion can be done during the first hepatectomy through the ligation and alcoholization of the right portal vein, which is the side more often embolized [71,72]. This modification is based on evidence that PVL triggers a similar or better regenerative response than PVE and could be safely applied, even in combination with partial hepatectomies of the left hemiliver.

In contemporary series of two-stage resection after PVE, 69% to 72% of the patients completed the second stage, the most common reason for dropout being tumour progression. Chemotherapy responsive patients who completed the resection have a 5-year survival rate of 32%-51% [73,74]. If new CLM or extrahepatic lesions are found, such as localized peritoneum implants, resection can still be performed if a R0 resection can be achieved. Pre-operative chemotherapy may be administered during the entire process.

Associating Liver Partition and Portal Vein Ligation for Staged Hepatectomy (ALPPS)

This technique has been recently described [75] It is a new concept of two-staged extended right hepatectomy with initial surgical exploration, right PVL, and in situ splitting (ISS) along the right side of the falciform ligament to induce rapid hypertrophy of the left lateral lobe in patients with marginally resectable or primarily nonresectable primary and metastatic liver tumours.

The selective embolization or ligation of segment IV portal branches when an extended right hepatectomy is planned has a significant impact on the hypertrophy of the FLR. However, the completeness of segment IV branch embolization requires optimal access and may frequently be incomplete. Combining PVL with ISS by nearly total parenchymal dissection induce a median hypertrophy of 74% (above that achieved by PVL or PVE alone) after a median time interval of 9 days.

This short time interval of about one week for hypertrophy overrides the risk of tumour progression in the meantime. Although for some patients the ALPPS can be the only chance to allow resection at all, further research needs to be conducted about short- and long-term results, such as accelerated development of micrometastases on the future remnant liver, systemic stress responses affecting the second step of resection, and survival and progression patterns [76]. In order to address the oncologic benefit of this new approach a registry has been created [77].

Laparoscopiy has also been used in this technique, showing that it is feasible and may be worthwhile in experienced hands [78,79].

Some authors have highlighted possible drawbacks of ALPPS such an increased morbidity and mortality rates in the first reported series [80], the presence a devascularized, necrotic segment 4 in patients who could not be candidates for second stage because of insuficient

http://dx.doi.org/10.5772/55898

hypertrophy [81] and scarce advantages over the previous techniques [82], recommending to reserve ALPPS for cases of unexpected tumour extension [83].

Technical advantages of ALPPS include an easier second procedure (the rapid hypertrophy of the remnant liver enables the second surgery before the development of adhesions), a faster recovery for the patient, with the possibility of restoring chemotherapy earlier, and the performance of the colorectal resection simultaneously with the first step of the procedure, including the tumour cleaning of the FLR (thus minimizing the risk of complications associated with postoperative liver failure) [84]. Of course, refinement in technical aspects and optimized patient selection for this procedure is needed (Figure 1).

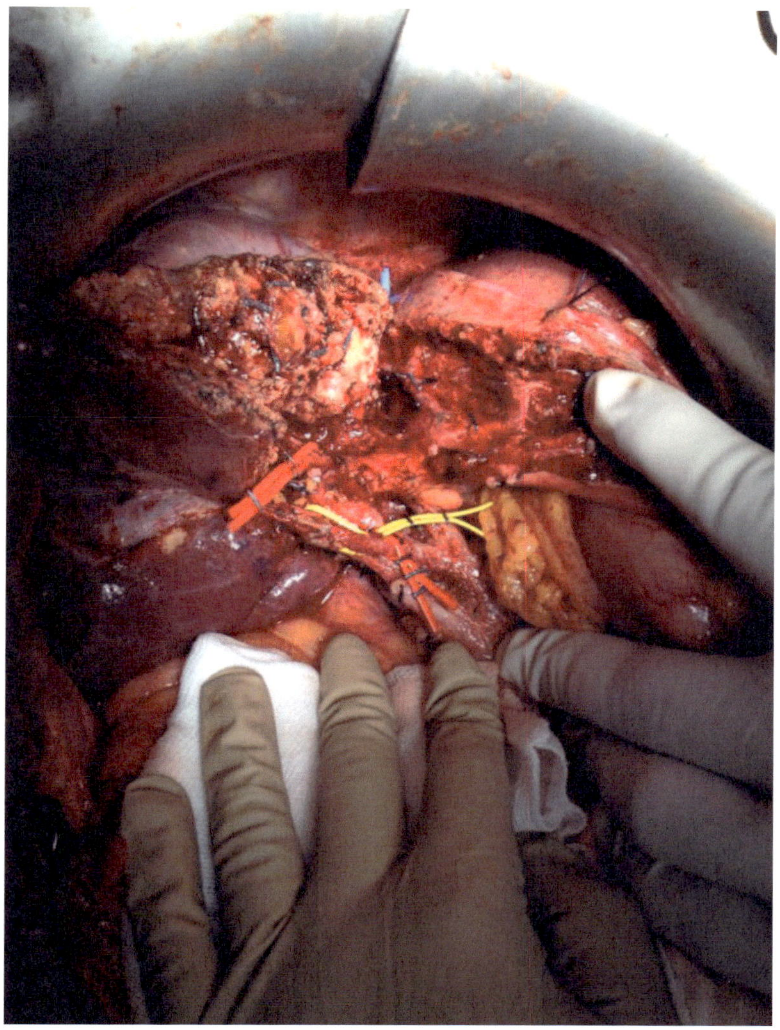

Figure 1. First stage of ALPPS

Ablative techniques

The precise role of ablative therapy is yet to be established. It can be used in patients with associated comorbidity that precludes resection and in patients who decline surgery, although there are significant risks associated with the procedure. Also patients with treatable extrahepatic disease or whose tumours have been downsized by chemotherapy but are not resectable may be considered for ablative therapy.

In radiofrequency ablation (RFA) a needle is placed into the centre of the metastasis. Alternating current results in frictional heat, which can reach up to 100°C, causing coagulative necrosis and irreversible tissue injury. The ablation zone varies in shape and size. Vessels situated next to the ablated tissue interfere with the ablative techniques by the "heat sink effect". Minor complications occur in 2.4 to 12% of patients; major complications appear in up to 5.6%; mortality rate is approximately 0.5% [85]. RFA treatment can achieve a 3-year survival rate of 25%. The combination of RFA and systemic chemotherapy has been shown to achieve a 5-year survival rate of 30% [86-88].

Laser-induced thermotherapy (LITT) consists in the local administration of laser light delivered to the tumour by means of fibers of quartz crystal. The heating effect destroys tissue. Morbidity and mortality are similar to RFA. Local tumour control at 6 months is achieved in approximately 97% of the patients [85].

For microwave ablation (MWA), microwaves are used to agitate water molecules in the tissue and produce frictional heat which leads to large volumes of coagulative necrosis. Transmission is not limited by tissue desiccation and charring as in RFA, allowing higher intratumoural temperatures, a larger ablation zone, shorter treatment time, and more complete tumour killing. Five-year survival rates of 32% have been reported.

High-intensity focused ultrasound (HIFU) is an innovative technique for the extracorporeal treatment of different tumour masses. Treatment is administered with a lens-focused transducer that elevates the tissue temperature to 60°C. In addition, the mechanical effects of the highintensity ultrasound assist the destruction of the tumour cells. Adverse effects seems to be minor [89].

Cryotherapy uses liquid nitrogen or argon to cool tumour tissue down to -180°C. The formation of intracellular ice crystals leads to a mechanical destruction of the interstitium. Cells on the borderline of the ablation zone are destroyed by dehydration and occlusion of small vessels. Repeating cycles of freezing and thawing are used to ensure irreversible cell damage. Complications are reported in approximately 30% of all cases. Mortality rates between 1.5% and 4%. An "ice-cracking" of the liver tissue is seen in 5 to 28% of the patients receiving the treatment. Five-year and 10-year survival rate of 44% and 19% are reported, respectively [90]. The increased local recurrence rates and the high complication rates have led to a diminishing use of this technique.

2.2.3. Total vascular exclusion: In-situ, ante-situ and ex-situ procedures

Techniques learned in liver transplantation, reduced adult-sized liver for children, living related donor liver transplantation and split liver transplantation are useful in liver resection.

Some tumours deemed unresectable with standard techniques can be resected using in-situ, ante-situ and ex-vivo or bench liver surgery.

The common basis for these techniques is the total vascular exclusion (TVE) of the liver and the perfusion of the organ by preservation hypothermic solution. The techniques differ in the extent to which liver is mobilized from its vascular connections, hilum and caval vein. Usually, veno-venous bypass is used to avoid venous congestion during prolonged caval and portal crossclamping and a hypothermic preservation solution is instilled through the portal vein. Hypothermic perfusion leads to a better tolerance to ischemia [91]. Wrapping of the liver with ice-cold towels is recommended to optimize the effect of cold preservation.

The main indications of the three techniques are tumours that involve vascular structures of the hylum, venous confluence or inferior vena cava (IVC), or are in close proximity to them. The technique to use depends on the tumour location and its relationship with the three hepatic veins and caval vein. In the ante-situ procedure the division of the suprahepatic vena cava allows rotation of the liver around the coronary axis, providing optimal exposition of the venous confluence and the retrohepatic vena cava. In the ex-situ technique the liver is completely removed from the patient and perfused with preservation solution, allowing complex reconstructions of hepatic veins or portal structures after which the liver is reimplanted. Since the first description by Pichlmayr in 1988, the technique has been sparingly applied in selected patients [92,93] due to its high morbidity and mortality.

The involvement of the IVC does not necessarily preclude resection since it can be resected and reconstructed with an autogenous vein graft or a prosthetic material. Morbidity and mortality rates (40% and 4.5-25%, respectively) appears to be balanced by the possible benefits, particularly when the lack of alternative approaches is considered [94].

2.2.4. Re-resection: Repeat hepatectomy

Recurrence may occur in up to 75% of CLM resected patients. About 70% of them are observed within the first 12 months after resection and 92% appear within 24 months [95]. Fifty percent of these relapses are in the liver [96] but only 5-27% of the patients are candidates for potentially curative repeated hepatectomy. Repeat hepatectomy is a safe and effective procedure under the same criteria of selection of the first hepatectomy. Although the prognostic variables provide rough indicators of prognosis, they should not be used as absolute contraindications to surgery. Each case needs a particular and specific evaluation: disease-free interval, number of metastases, quality of life, general health condition, resectable extrahepatic disease, assessment of residual liver volume, etc. by the multidisciplinary team.

Recurrence after repeat hepatectomy has been reported in 60–80% of patients [97]. Some patients have resectable disease limited to the liver and may be candidates for a third or even fourth hepatic resection.

Between 9% and 30% of patients with a second hepatectomy for CLM have a third resection [2,98-100] and around 4% of them have a fourth resection [101].

The safety of multiple repeated hepatic resections has been demonstrated, with a low mortality rate (0%-2%) and a morbidity rate of 5%-30%, not significantly different from those who have had only one or two liver resections. LiverMet Survey published the largest series (n = 251) of third hepatectomies for recurrent CLM showing a survival benefit of 29% at 5 years. Technically, re-hepatectomies are more difficult than the first procedure because of dense adhesions and because the liver parenchyma may be more fibrotic or friable.

3. Non-colorectal liver metastases

Pancreas, breast, ovary, rectum and stomach are the following sources of liver metastasis after those of colonic origin in decreasing order of frequency [102]. Liver metastases from colorectal cancer have a less aggressive clinical and biological behavior than those from others solid tumours, like breast or lung, in which the liver is another site of systemic disease [103].

3.1. Liver metastases for neuroendocrine tumours

Gastrointestinal neuroendocrine tumours (NETs) are a diverse group of tumours that originate throughout the gastrointestinal tract and are characterized by a relative slow growth rate and the potential to produce and secret a variety of hormones. NETs can be classified into carcinoid and pancreatic histological subtypes. NETs of pancreatic origin can be non-functioning or can produce hormonally active substances: insulin, gastrin, vasoactive intestinal peptide. Carcinoid tumours arise commonly in the midgut and may secret serotonin and other bioactive amines.

Most of NETs will have diseminated disease at the time of diagnosis, with a 5-year survival between 50% and 80%. The liver is the most common organ involved, followed by bone and lung [104]. Almost 10% of all liver metastases are neuroendocrine in origin. The presence of liver metastases of NETs (LMNETs) is a distinguishing feature of malignant neuroendocrine tumours and is the rate-limiting step for patient's survival [105]. LMNETs occur in 50% to 75% of small-bowel carcinoids, in 5% to 70% of foregut carinoids and about 14% of hindgut carcinoids. Furthermore, in many patients the liver remains the only site of metastatic disease for a prolonged period of time. Usually LMNETs are multifocal, bilobar and in more than half of the cases involve more than 50% of the liver parenchyma [106]. In spite of it, Hodul et al concluded that hepatic resection resulted in an almost double 5-year survival rate compared with the non-resected group (47-82% vs. 30-40%, respectively) [107].

Management of LMNETs is challenging, since there is not a firm consensus on the optimal treatment strategy, except the Steimueller's guidelines [108,109] (Table 1).

Several studies have shown 5-year survival rates of up to 85% in R0 resection for both primary and secondary sites (Table 2). Cytoreduction is usefull as a palliative approach but it needs to reache at least 90% of tumour volume reduction to improve both survival and symptoms [110].

Table 2: Liver resection for neuroendocrine liver metastases

1. LMNET without extrahepatic disease:

a Preferred treatment: surgical resection of both primary and all liver metastasis ± local ablative techniques (may be one or two-step procedure)

b Treatment if unresectable disease or poor surgical candidate: continued biotherapy, hepatic artery chemoembolization (TACE) or embolization and RFA

c Liver transplantation considered in rare cases (less than 1%)

2. LMNET with extrahepatic disease:

a Preferred treatment: biotherapy or other systemic nonsurgical treatment

b Palliative treatment if symptoms progress:

- If small number of isolated liver metastases less than 3-4 cm: RFA, TACE or embolization; may consider minor or anatomic resection in selected cases
- If complex pattern or liver metastases: RFA, or embolization; may consider major liver resection together with RFA for selected cases
- If diffuse pattern of liver metastases: TACE or embolization

Table 1. Consensus guidelines for the treatment of liver metastases from endocrine tumours:

Authors	Year	# of patients	Resolution of symptoms (%)	Survival (%)
Sarmiento et al [110]	2003	170	96	75 at 3 years; 61 at 5 years
Knox et al [111]	2003	13	82	85 at 5 years
Touzios et al [106]	2005	19	95	72 at 5 years
Musunuru et [112]	2006	13	100	83 at 3 years

Table 2. Liver resection for neuroendocrine liver metastases

After surgery, the normalization of tumour markers, 5-hydroxyindoleacetic acid (5-HIAA) and chromogranin A predict a complete resection. This last marker is more sensitive than 5-HIAA to diagnose progression or recurrence.

RFA has been used as the sole method to achieve relief of symptoms and local control. Although this goal is attained in 60% to 80% of cases of LMNETs, a sustained response rate is low.

TACE is contraindicated when the tumour size exceeds 50% of the liver due to the risk of liver failure. The duration of response is short and here is also a risk of causing carcinoid tumour lysis syndrome or crises.

Several authors advocate liver and multivisceral transplant in unresectable LMNETs, but the role of liver transplantation in patients with LMNETs remains controversial, especially given the shortage of donors. Less than 1% of all liver transplants have been performed for LMNETs and, outside of a few small studies, survival does not seem to have improved. Frilling et al suggested a set of criteria for transplantation of patients with LMNETs: age younger than 65, primary tumour under control, absence of extrahepatic disease proven over a 6-month period, progression of liver tumours and excessive hormonal symptoms refractory to medical therapy [113].

An aggressive surgical approach using multi.modality therapy (resection, embolization and RFA) leads to long-term survival in these patients. Although long-term cure can only be achieved in a small proportion of patients with malignant NETs, significant long-term palliation can be achieved. This aggressive surgical approach can be recommended, keeping in mind that additional liver-directed procedures may be required or combined with surgery to achieve effectiveness for a good quality of life.

3.2. Non-colorectal non-neuroendocrine liver metastases

Despite the established agreement on the advantage of liver resection for metastatic colorectal and neuroendocrine tumours, the role of hepatic surgery in patients with liver metastases from non-colorectal non-neuroendocrine (NCRNNE) carcinoma is not well defined. However, the results reported in a number of recent studies support a developing trend toward surgery in this setting.

There are many reasons for this lack of clear-sightedness. Because of these ununiformed characteristics, the conclusions are that prognostic factors for liver metastases from NCRNNE remain uncertain. These is due to many reports include neuroendocrine tumour patients in their analysis and consequently alter survival data. In fact, most series are not comparable in terms of mid- and long-term (tumour-free) survival, as they include patients with NCRNNE hepatic metastases from different primary malignancies, different frequency of isolated hepatic metastases and different tumoural behaviour, different sensitivity to chemotherapy and different length of disease-free interval between the resection of the primary tumour and the diagnosis of the liver metastases. In addition, to influence the variability of the series, many studies include recruitment periods of 10 years or more so the chemotherapy regime has been changed a lot and the results should be taken with caution.

In recent years, despite the poor results, liver resection for metastases suitable for surgery have been carried out. The main reasons for this attitude have been above-mentioned. Also, there are no data that actually suggest the usefulness of alternative treatments for NCRNNE liver metastases, so this reinforces the role of surgery.

The aggressive policy used by some surgeons and oncologists, in relation to metastases confined to the liver, should be moderated considering generic variables, such as disease-free interval from the primary tumour. Twelve months is considered as the generic minimum period between primary tumour and secondary disease to give an indication for surgery for liver metastases. After this first year, any further time interval should be considered as a progressively increasing positive prognostic factor. A longer disease-free interval is believed to indicate less aggressive tumour biology or less account of tumoural stem-cells [103]. In a retrospective study of 1452 patients treated at 41 centres, Adam et al demonstrated that liver resection for NCRNNE hepatic metastases is safe and effective (Table 3). The authors categorized the outcome according to the primary tumour and the 5-year survival after liver resection into: favorable (adrenal, testicular, ovarian, small bowel, ampullary, breast, renal, and uterine tumours); intermediate (gastric adenocarcinoma, exocrine pancreas, cutaneous melanoma, choroidal melanoma, and duodenal tumours); and poor (gastroesophageal junction, pulmonary, esophageal, and head and neck tumours) [114].

Author	Years	# of patients	5 years survival
Harrison LE 1997 [116]	1980-1995	96	37%
Hemming AW 2000 [117]	1978-1998	37	45%
Laurent C 2001 [118]	1980-1997	39	35%
Yamada H 2001 [119]	1990-1995	33	12.1%
Takada Y 2001 [120]	1987-1999	14	NR
Karavias DD 2002 [121]	1994-2001	18	NR
Weitz J 2005 [122]	1981-2002	141	57%*
Ercolani G 2005 [123]	NS	142	34.3%
Adam R 2006 [114]	1983-2004	1452	36%

Table 3. Studies with NCNNE liver metastases resection

The role of liver resection for NCRNNE liver metastases is still a matter of discussion because only small studies have been carried out in this field and the conclusive outcomes are collective and not specific for each type of tumour. In a comparative analysis, Reddy et al studied the results of liver resection for metastatic tumours in 360 consecutive patients (245 colorectal and 33 neuroendocrine versus 82 NCRNNE primaries). There were no difference in median overall survival between patients with metastases from colorectal and noncolorectal disease. The long-term outcome after resection of NCRNNE was nearly equivalent to that of colorectal tumours [115].

3.2.1. Gastrointestinal stromal tumours liver metastases

Gastrointestinal stromal tumours (GIST) are the most common mesenchymal neoplasms of the gastrointestinal tract and account for 1%-3% of all gastrointestinal malignancies [124]. It is thought that these tumours differentiate from intestinal pacemaker cells, also known as interstitial cells of Cajal [125,126]. They affect mostly males between the ages of 50 and 70, and are usually found incidentally at early stages. Large or advanced lesions may present with a variety of clinical findings, including bleeding, abdominal pain, early satiety, bowel obstruction or perforation.

The only definitive treatment for GIST is surgical resection. These tumours demonstrate a broad spectrum of biological behaviours, from indolent to rapidly progressive malignancies [127]. The liver is known to be a common metastatic site for GIST and previous studies have reported that 55%-72% of patients develop hepatic metastasis following complete resection of the primary tumour [128]. Previously described treatment modalities for hepatic metastases from GIST include anthracycline and ifosfamide-based chemotherapy regimes, TACE, surgical resection and hepatic transplantation. However, high recurrence rates and poor survival outcomes following hepatic transplantation have been reported. Radical surgical resection, including hepatectomy, is the only potential treatment modality for this clinical condition. Liver resection itself has been shown to prolong survival; this seems especially true for patients with small metastasis and a long disease-free interval. A time to metastasis of 2 years has actually been an independent predictor of outcome in a large group of patients with a median survival of 61 months [129].

Imatinib mesylate (Glivec®), a selective inhibitor of tyrosine kinase, has revolutionized the management of this disease in recent years. Imatinib has a significant shrinking effect on GIST and can be used when primary GIST have attained a very large size or are in unfavorable locations, increasing the risk of positive resection margins [125]. Imatinib has also become the first line of treatment for recurrent and/or metastatic GIST. Before the advent of tyrosine kinase inhibitors (TKIs), surgical resection was the primary treatment for hepatic gastrointestinal stromal tumour (GIST) metastases. Although TKIs have improved survival in the metastatic setting, outcomes after multimodal therapy comprised of hepatectomy and TKIs for GIST are unknown. A recent report concludes that combination therapy for GIST liver metastases comprised of surgical resection and TKIs therapy is more effective than surgery or TKIs therapy alone [130]. There are significant prognostic implications in GIST cases with hepatic metastasis. Recent studies have shown an overall median survival time of 39 (33-40) months following surgery. Resection of GIST liver metastases may be curative when the primary disease has been eradicated and negative surgical resection margins are attained (Table 4).

Author	Years	# of patients	Median survival (months)	Recurrence (months)
Ng [131]	1957–1987	5	33	Not recorded
Chen et al. [132]	1984–1995	6	39	3 (50%)
Lang et al. [133]	1983–1996	18	40	9 (60%)
DeMatteo et al. [128]	1982–1998	56	39	47 (84%)
[134]l.	1989–2001	10	39	7 (70%)
[135]	1984–2003	18	36	14 (77%)
Gomez et al. [127]	1993– 2005	12	43	8 (73%)

Table 4. Surgical resection for hepatic metastases from GIST, sarcomas and leiomyosarcomas

Surgical resection with curative intent for hepatic metastases from GIST should be considered when feasible, as it may improve survival outcomes in selected patients. Recurrence of disease can be managed with further surgery, RFA, imatinib mesylate therapy or a combination of these treatment modalities.

http://dx.doi.org/10.5772/55898

3.2.2. *Liver Metastases from Breast Cancer (LMBC)*

Patients with visceral metastases from breast cancer have an unlucky prognosis. Liver metastases are infrequent as the sole site of systemic disease and even rarer as a solitary metastasis. Only 3% to 11% of the patients have the liver as the single involved organ out of 65% of breast cancer patients with liver metastases as part of the disseminated disease [136]. Although systemic treatment can achieve response in around 60% of patients, long-term survival is unusual, varying from 1 to 15 months [137]. Moreover, around 70% of these liver metastases are negative for hormonal receptors so that chemotherapy is usually the only treatment.

Extrahepatic disease has been considered as a contraindication for liver resection in these patients, but some reports have not found differences in survival between operated patients with or without extrahepatic breast cancer metastases, bearing in mind that most of the these extrahepatic lesions were bone metastases treated with chemotherapy and radiotherapy previously to surgery [138]. This retrospective study of 454 patients operated on for metastatic breast cancer reported that 41 and 21% of these patients remain alive at 5 and 10 years, respectively.

Few series of liver resection have been published [139,140], describing around 250 patients operated in a few highly specialized centers (Table 5).

Autor	N	Solitary Metastasis	5 years Survival Rate	Pronostic factors
Sakamoto et al (2005) [141]	34	19/34	21	extrahepatic diseases
Carlini et al (2002) [142]	17	15/17	46	
Yoshimoto et al (2000)[143]	25	14/25	27	"/> 1 year
Selzner et al (2000) [144]	17		22	"/> 4 years
Pocard et al (2001)[145]	65	44/65	46	N0
Seifert et al (1999)[136]	15		53(3 years)	R0
Raab et al (1996)[146]	34	21/35	18	Local Recurrence
Scheuerlein et al (1998)[147]	21	9 of 21	60(2 years)	R0

Table 5. Liver resection from breast cancer

These differences among series in outcome following hepatic resection may merely reflect difference in selection criteria and in tumour biology. Resection criteria for liver metastases from breast cancer are not yet clearly defined and a number of questions remain to be answered: Must hepatectomy be done in patients with extrahepatic disease? Which chemotherapy regimens must be given before and after surgery? Which is the best timing for liver surgery?

Eighty percent of the liver metastases were due to primary tumours less than 5 cm in size and the number of patients with a solitary metastasis varied from 41% to 79%. The lapse of time between breast surgery and diagnosis of the liver lesions was 21 to 60 months [140,145].

Reponse to chemotherapy appears to be an important predictor of survival following hepatic resection for liver metastases from breast cancer. In the Adam paper, patients who remained stable or progressed on prehepatectomy chemotherapy were 3.5 times more likely to die than responders. Indeed, preoperative chemotherapy is a modality to prolong survival and the response can be considered as a selection criteria.

Two pronostic factors have been identified by several authors [145]: prolonged tumour-free interval (1-2 years) between breast cancer surgery and liver metastases diagnosis and no lymph node involvement at the time of breast cancer. Liver surgery should be offered to every patient with a good performance status, with predictable R0 resection and with a long disease-free interval (Figure 2).

In synchronous tumours, disease must be stabilized with chemotherapy. To consider surgery, there should not be extrahepatic disease or it must be a solitary bone metastasis. Surgery can be technically hampered because of the effects of chemotherapy on liver parenchyma. Hillar lymphadenectomy can be considered since positive lymph nodes are frequent, although they do not exclude resection.

Liver recurrence is very high but the best chemotherapy regimen in these cases is to be defined. Survival after resection is longer compared with other treatments, although disease-free time is usually brief.

Other studies suggest that liver resection in highly selected patients may function as a cytoreductive rather than a curative procedure, because breast liver metastases is considered as a disseminated disease, but as a cytoreductive approach it improves the survival rate.

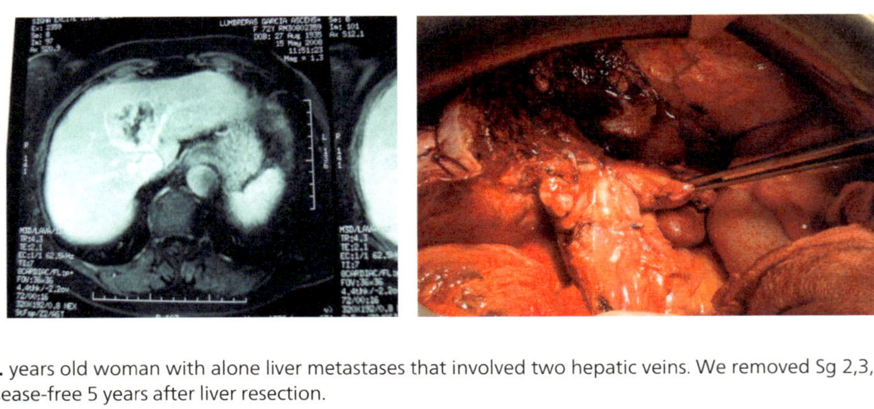

Figure 2. years old woman with alone liver metastases that involved two hepatic veins. We removed Sg 2,3,4,5,and 8. She is disease-free 5 years after liver resection.

3.2.3. Liver metastases from melanoma

Up to 30% of patients with melanoma develop distant metastases. After the luns and brain, the liver is the third most involved organ. Previously considered an infrequent condition, autopsy studies have shown liver metastases in 55%-75% of the patients with melanoma [148,149]. Diagnosis is generally made by imaging studies during follow-up, since symptoms are suggestive of advanced disease. FDG PET/CT shows a sensitivity of 85%, a specificity of 100% and a positive predictive value of 98% [150]. Median survival in these patients ranges between 2 and 6 months [151]. Palliative radiotherapy and systemic chemotherapy do not prolong survival and, although interferon-α and interleukin-2 have yielded promising response rates, these are rarely durable [152].

Liver resection achieves 5-year survival rate between 5% and 25% [153] (Table 6). A reduction in immunosuppressive factors and a slowing of the growth of occult metastases have been proposed as part of the beneficial effects of surgery [154]. A large series reports a 21% 5-year survival rate for 104 patients after resection of liver metastases from melanoma of choroidal origin and a 22% 5-year survival rate for 44 patients with the same condition but with a cutaneous source [114]. The same paper confirmed that choroid melanomas were commonly associated with multiple intrahepatic tumours but were less likely than cutaneous melanomas to be associated with extrahepatic disease. A series collected from four centres showed that the location of the primary tumour substantially impacts on the recurrence and survival after resection of secondary liver tumours. Among 40 patients who underwent liver resection, the rate of recurrent hepatic metastases was higher among patients with ocular (53.3%) compared to those with cutaneous tumours (17.4%) [148].

Authors	Year	n	5-year survival (%)	Median survival (months)
Ripley et al. [155]	2010	35	53	-
Rose et al. [149]	2001	24	29	28
Pawlik et al. [148]	2006	24	47.2(2years)	23.6
Chua et al. [153]	2010	13	40 (3years)	21
Herman et al. [156]	2007	10	-	22
Crook et al. [157]	2006	5	-	-

Table 6. Liver resection in melanoma

Positive prognostic factors are a R0 resection, a solitary metastasis and absence of extrahepatic disease [155]. Resection with negative margins offers the only chance of long-term survival, since for R1 and R2 resection there are not periods of survival longer than 6 months.

For all the authors, liver resection must not be considered as a curative treatment but as a part of the whole oncologic treatment because of its cytoreductive nature. Reported series during the last decade show that liver resection of metastases from melanoma are infrequent, that the interval between treatment of primary and secondary tumour is long (49 to 96 months), that mayor hepatectomies are performed in 50% to 60% of the patients and that survival varies widely (0% to 53%), which indicates that this is a very heterogeneous group of patients with a very variable criteria for resection.

3.2.4. *Liver metastases from gastric cancer and others non-colorectal gastrointestinal adenocarcinoma*

Many reports defend liver resection for metastatic gastric cancer although the indications for resection have not been established. Frequently, liver metastases suggest an advance disease with a mean survival of less than 6 month. Last studies showed increased survival benefit with 5-year survivors between 20%-42%.

Positive pronostic factors have been indentified: solitary tumour or no more than 3 nodules, size less than 5 cm, unilobular distribution, resection margin more than 10 mm and disease-free interval between gastric cancer resection and liver metastases longer than 1 year [158]. In a study by Thelen the multivariate analysis revealed only resection margin as an independent prognostic factor for survival [159]. Shirabe concluded that synchronous hepatectomy should not be a contraindication for hepatic resection [160] (Table 7).

Authors	Year	n	5-year survival (%)
Ambiru et al. [161]	2001	40	15
Zacherl et al. [162]	2002	15	0
Saiura et al. [163]	2002	10	20
Okano et al. [164]	2002	19	21
Shirabe et al. [160]	2003	36	11
Sakamoto et al. [158]	2003	26	4
Roh et al. [165]	2005	11	18
Summary		157	12,1

Table 7. long-term of liver resection in gastric cancer

In conclusion, the results of liver resection in liver gastric metastases should not be dismissed simply because there is not prospective, randomized data. For patients with hepatic disease amenable to surgical resection, treatment alternatives include systemic chemotherapy, locoregional ablative therapies with or without systemic treatment or surgical resection with or without systemic treatment. It is not unreasonable to consider liver resections in highly selected patients as part of multidisciplinary care for this malignancy.

For other non-colorectal gastrointestinal adenocarcinoma the available evidence for hepatectomy is extremely limited, and this treatment strategy lacks utility. Most authors, despite having performed hepatectomies for these metastatic tumours, agree that it is associated with a poor prognosis.

3.2.5. *Liver metastases from lung cancer*

We can re-emphasize that the refinements in perioperative care and surgical techniques have significantly improved the safety of liver surgery, and operative mortality has decreased to around 1% in tertiary referring centres. For this, in the last 10 years liver resection has been proposed not only for colorectal and neuroendocrine metastases, but also for metastatic tumour from other sites such as lung cancer.

Liver resection for lung cancer metastases are rare and few number of cases are reported in the literature. The reported cases appear frequently with other kind of metastastic liver tumour in more large series. Lindlell et al., in the largest serie, reported three cases but did not show the outcome [166]. Di Carlo reported a case of long-term survival [167].

In summary, when a patient has one or two liver nodules with more than one year of disease-free interval from the resection of primary tumour, hepatic resection can be a therapeutic option [168]. Liver involvement is managed surgically only under these exceptional circumstances.

3.2.6. Liver metastases from ovarian and testicular cancer

Epithelial ovarian cancer is a highly chemosensitive disease, and platinum-based therapies bring about significant diminution of tumour volume in most of the patients. Regrettably, the patients develop resistance to platinum chemotherapy after 24-36 months. Notwithstanding, many centres, despite stage III-IV advanced ovarian cancer, with a median survival of 3.5 years, propose very aggressive management with surgical debulking [169]. Five-years disease-specific survival after hepatic resection in patients with hepatic metastases from NCRNNE carcinoma is comparable to the 5-year survival of patients after hepatic resection for colorectal cancer, ranging from 9% to 38%, depending on the type of primary tumour. For this, multiple studies have shown an important survival benefit when primary cytoreductive surgery precedes the initiation of chemotherapy for advanced ovarian cancer. The benefits of cytoreductive surgery are also obvious in patients with recurrent disease. More than 70% of patients with advanced stage disease suffer recurrence and the benefits of second debulking depend on chemosensitivity, feasibility of surgery and tumour behaviour.

The liver is rarely the only site of metastatic ovarian cancer but also hepatectomy can be important in a cytoreduction approach. Ovarian cancer can involve the liver through peritoneal lesions on the surface or with intraparenchymal metastases [170]. Survival is clearly improved for stage IV disease patients with complete and adequate debulking, even hepatectomy.

In conclusion, hepatic metastases should not preclude attempts at optimal secondary cytoreductive surgery. When cytoreductive resection is performed by pelvic and hepatobiliary surgeons, morbidity and mortality appear no different from that attributed to aggressive surgical debulking istself.

Metastasectomy is wel established in the management of disseminated non-seminomatous germ cell testicular carcinoma that does not completely respond to chemotherapy. Testicular cancer has often been described as 'the model of a curable cancer'. Previously to the mid-1970s treatment cured less than 5% of patients; by 1984, the cure rate for testicular cancer was higher 80% and experimental protocols began to focus on the refractory cases or 'poor risk' patients. The key to success in the treatment of metastatic germ cell tumours is due to the multidisciplinary approach. Although after chemotherapy it can be difficult to differentiate active residual tumour from necrosis or fibrosis, the probability of achieving cure by surgical resection is high. For these reasons, lymphadenectomy and visceral resection are recommended if there is imaging evidence of residual disease [171]. In some cases complete excision requires multivisceral radical resections as a last attempt to cure patients who have exhausted all other therapeutic options. Complete surgical resection of all measurable disease is the gold standard and correlates with improvement in both relapse-free and overall survival after hepatectomy, with actuarial survival rates of 78% at 3 years in these tumours.

3.2.7. Renal cell carcinoma and urothelial cancer

The available data on hepatic resection for renal cell cancer (RCC) metastases and urothelial cancer (UC) are limited to case reports. In metastatic RCC, the liver involvement is present in 20% of the patients and carries less than 10% of overall 1-year survival rate. Furthermore, only 5% of metastatic RCC patients have the liver as only involved organ. However, five-year survival of 33% has been reported following resection of lung, brain or lymph node metastases in association with chemotherapy in UC. Furthermore, metastasectomy has been used for palliation with good results [171]. However Alves et al. reported 46 liver resection for metastatic RCC patients with a 5-year survival of 13% [172].

These limited data determine inconsistent recommendations for hepatectomy in metastatic RCC and UC. In RCC, the use of sunitinib or surafenib as neoadjuvant or post-hepatectmy therapy could improve the outcome.

Author details

Alejandro Serrablo[1*], Luis Tejedor[2] and Jose-Manuel Ramia[3]

*Address all correspondence to: almaley@telefonica.net

1 Hepatopancreatic biliary Surgical Unit, Miguel Servet University Hospital, Zaragoza, Spain

2 General Surgery Service, Punta de Europa Hospital, Algeciras, Spain

3 Hepatopancreatic biliary Surgical Unit, Guadalajara University Hospital, Guadalajara, Spain

References

[1] Hugh, T. J, Ghaneh, P, & Poston, G. J. Hepatic metastases. In: Garden OJ (ed.) Hepatobiliary and Pancreatic Surgery. Philadelphia: Elsevier Saunders; (2005)., 97-130.

[2] Fong, Y, Fortner, J, Sun, R. L, Brennan, M. F, & Blumgart, L. H. Clinical score for predicting recurrence after hepatic resection metastatic colorectal cancer: analysis of 1001 consecutive cases. Ann Surg (1999). , 230, 309-18.

[3] Nordlinger, B, Guiguet, M, Vaillant, J. C, Balladur, P, Boudjema, K, & Bachellier, P. Surgical resection of colorectal carcinoma metastases to the liver. A prognostic scoring system to improve case selection, based on 1568 patients. Cancer (1996). , 77, 1254-62.

[4] Rees, M, Tekkis, P. P, Welsh, F. K, Rourke, O, & John, T. TG. Evaluation of long-term survival after hepatic resection for metastatic colorectal cancer: a multifactorial model of 929 patients. Ann Surg (2008). , 247, 125-35.

[5] Zakaria, S, Donohue, J. H, Que, F. G, Farnell, M. B, Schleck, C. D, Ilstrup, D. M, & Nagorney, D. M. Hepatic resection for colorectal metastases: value for risk scoring systems? Ann Surg (2007). , 246, 183-91.

[6] Iwatsuki, S, Dvorchik, I, Madariaga, J. R, Marsh, J. W, Dodson, F, Bonham, A. C, Geller, D. A, Gayowsky, T. J, Fung, J. J, & Starzl, T. E. Hepatic resection for metastatic colorectal adenocarcinoma: a proposal of a prognostic scoring system. J Am Coll Surg (1999). , 189, 291-9.

[7] Adam, R, Wicherts, D. A, De Haas, R. J, et al. Patients with initially unresectable colorectal liver metastases: is there a possibility of cure? J Clin Oncol (2009). , 27, 1829-35.

[8] El Khodary, M, Milot, L, & Reinhold, C. Imaging of Hepatic Metastases. In: Brodt P (ed.) Liver Metastasis: Biology and Clinical Management. New York: Springer Science+Business Media B.978-9-40070-291-2, 2011, 307-353.

[9] Kinkel, K, Lu, Y, Both, M, Warren, R. S, & Thoeni, R. F. (2002). Detection of hepatic metastases from cancers of the gastrointestinal tract by using noninvasive imaging methods (US, CT, MR Imaging, PET): a meta-analysis. Radiology 2002;, 224, 748-56.

[10] Chami, L, Lassau, N, Malka, D, Ducreux, M, Bidault, S, Roche, A, & Elias, D. Benefits of Contrast-Enhanced Sonography for the Detection of Liver Lesions: Comparison with Histologic Findings. AJR (2008). , 190, 683-90.

[11] Larsen LPSRole of contrast enhanced ultrasonography in the assessment of hepatic metastases: A review. World J Hepatol (2012). , 2(1), 8-15.

[12] Guglielmi, A, Pachera, S, & Ruzzenente, A. Surgical Therapy of Hepatic Metastases. In: Delaini GG (ed.) Rectal Cancer: New Frontiers in Diagnosis, Treatment and Rehabilitation. Milan: Springer-Verlag; (2005). , 227-241.

[13] Laghi, A, Sansoni, I, Celestre, M, Paolantonio, P, & Passariello, R. Computed Tomography. In: Lencioni R, Cioni D, Bartolozzi C (eds.) Focal Liver Lesions Detection, Characterization, Ablation. Berlin Heidelberg: Springer-Verlag; (2005). , 17-32.

[14] Yang, S, Ho, S, Hanna, S. S, Gallinger, S, Wei, A. C, Kiss, A, & Law, C. Utility of preoperative imaging in evaluating colorectal liver metastases declines over time. HPB (2010). , 12(9), 605-9.

[15] Bluemke, D. A, Paulson, E. K, Choti, M. A, Desena, S, & Clavien, P. A. Detection of Hepatic Lesions in Candidates for Surgery: Comparison of Ferumoxides-Enhanced MR Imaging and Dual-Phase Helical CT. AJR (2000). , 175, 1653-58.

[16] Vidiri, A, Carpanese, L, Annibale, D, Caterino, M, Cosimelli, M, Zeuli, M, David, M, & Crecco, V. M. Evaluation of Hepatic Metastases from Colorectal Carcinoma with MR-Superparamagnetic Iron Oxide. J Exp Clin Cancer Res (2004). , 23(1), 53-60.

[17] Koh, D. M, Scurr, E, Collins, D. J, Pirgon, A, Kanber, B, Karanjia, N, Brown, G, Leach, M. O, & Husband, J. E. Colorectal hepatic metastases: quantitative measurements using single-shot echo-planar diffusion-weighted MR imaging. Eur Radiol (2006). , 16, 1898-905.

[18] Koike, N, Cho, A, Nasu, K, Seto, K, Nagaya, S, Ohshima, Y, & Ohkohchi, N. Role of diffusion-weighted magnetic resonance imaging in the differential diagnosis of focal hepatic lesions. World J Gastroenterol (2009). , 15(46), 5805-12.

[19] Udayasankar, U, Chamsuddin, A, Mittal, P, & Small, W. C. Diagnostic imaging and image-guided interventions of hepatobiliary malignancies. In: Blake MA, Kalra MK (eds.) Imaging in Oncology. New York: Springer Science+Business Media, LLC; (2008). , 199-228.

[20] Valls, C, Martinez, L, Ruiz, S, & Alba, E. Radiological imaging of liver metastases. In: Vauthey JN, Hoff PMG, Audisio RA, Poston GJ (eds.) Liver metastases. London: Springer-Verlag; (2009). , 1-13.

[21] Bipat, S, Van Leeuwen, M. S, Comans, E. F, Pijl, M. E, Bossuyt, P. M, Zwinderman, A. H, & Stoker, J. Colorectal liver metastases: CT, MR imaging, and PET for diagnosis-metaanalysis. Radiology (2005). , 237, 123-31.

[22] Wiering, B. Krabbe PFM, Jager GJ, Oyen WJG, Ruers TJF. The Impact of Fluor-18-Deoxyglucose-Positron Emission Tomography in the Management of Colorectal Liver Metastases: A Systematic Review and Metaanalysis. Cancer (2005). , 104(12), 2658-70.

[23] Patel, S, Mccall, M, Ohinmaa, A, Bigam, D, & Dryden, D. M. Positron emission tomography/computed tomographic scans compared to computed tomographic scans for detecting colorectal liver metastases: a systematic review. Ann Surg (2011). , 253(4), 666-71.

[24] Niekel, M. C. Bipat Sh, Stoker J. Diagnostic Imaging of Colorectal Liver Metastases with CT, MR Imaging, FDG PET, and/or FDG PET/CT: A Meta-Analysis of Prospective Studies Including Patients Who Have Not Previously Undergone Treatment. Radiology (2010). , 257(3), 674-84.

[25] Sørensen, M, Mortensen, F. V, Høyer, M, Vilstrup, H, & Keiding, S. and The Liver Tumour Board at Aarhus University Hospital. FDG-PET improves management of

patients with colorectal liver metastases allocated for local treatment: a consecutive prospective study. Scand J Surg (2007). , 96, 209-13.

[26] Pawlik, T, Assumpcao, L, Vossen, J, Buijs, M, Gleisner, A, Schulick, R, & Choti, M. Trends in nontherapeutic laparotomy rates in patients undergoing surgical therapy for hepatic colorectal metastases. Ann Surg Oncol (2009). , 16(2), 371-78.

[27] Fernandez, F. G, Drebin, J. A, Linehan, D. C, Dehdashti, F, Siegel, B. A, & Strasberg, S. M. Fiveyear survival after resection of hepatic metastases from colorectal cancer in patients screened by positron emission tomography with F-18 fluorodeoxyglucose (FDGPET). Ann Surg (2004). , 240(3), 438-50.

[28] Fioole, B, De Haas, R. J, Wicherts, D. A, Elias, S. G, Scheffers, J. M, Van Hillegersberg, R, & Van Leeuwen, M. S. Borel Rinkes IH. Additional value of contrast enhanced intraoperative ultrasound for colorectal liver metastases. Eur J Radiol (2008). , 67(1), 169-76.

[29] Leen, E, Ceccotti, P, Moug, S. J, & Glen, P. MacQuarrie J, Angerson WJ, Albrecht T, Hohmann J, Oldenburg A, Ritz JP, Horgan PG. Potential value of contrast-enhanced intraoperative ultrasonography during partial hepatectomy for metastases: an essential investigation before resection? Ann Surg (2006). , 243, 236-40.

[30] Nakano, H, Ishida, Y, Hatakeyama, T, Sakuraba, K, Hayashi, M, Sakurai, O, & Hataya, K. Contrast-enhanced intraoperative ultrasonography equipped with late Kupffer-phase image obtained by sonazoid in patients with colorectal liver metastases. World J Gastroenterol (2008). , 14(20), 3207-11.

[31] Torzilli, G. Del Fabbro D, Palmisano A, Donadon M, Bianchi P, Roncalli M, Balzarini L, Montorsi M. Contrast-enhanced intraoperative ultrasonography during hepatectomies for colorectal cancer liver metastases. J Gastrointest Surg (2005). , 9, 1148-53.

[32] Bipat, S, & Van Leeuwen, M. S. IJzermans JNM, Comans EFI, Planting AST, Bossuyt PMM, Greve J-W, Stoker J. Evidence-based guideline on management of colorectal liver metastases in the Netherlands. Ned J Med (2007). , 63(1), 1-14.

[33] Doan, P. L, Vauthey, J. N, Palavecino, M, & Morse, M. A. Colorectal Liver Metastases. In: Clavien PA, Breitenstein S (eds.) Malignant Liver Tumours. Current and Emerging Therapies. Oxford: Wiley-Blackwell; (2012). , 342-346.

[34] Vauthey, J. N. The AHPBA (2006). Consensus Conference: Focus on Improving Resectability in Patients With Hepatic Colorectal Metastases. Medscape Oncology 2006. http://www.medscape.org/viewarticle/524135accessed 27 August 2012)

[35] Foster, J. H. Survival after liver resection for secondary tumours. Am J Surg (1978). , 135, 389-94.

[36] Kopetz, S, Chang, G. J, Overman, M. J, Eng, C, Sargent, D. J, Larson, D. W, Grothey, A, Vauthey, J. N, Nagorney, D. M, & Mcwilliams, R. R. Improved survival in meta-

static colorectal cancer is associated with adoption of hepatic resection and improved chemotherapy. J Clin Oncol (2009). , 27, 3677-83.

[37] Altendorf-hofmann, A, & Scheele, J. A critical review of the major indicators of prognosis after resection of hepatic metastases from colorectal carcinoma. Surg Oncol Clin N Am (2003). , 12, 165-92.

[38] Figueras, J, Burdio, F, Ramos, E, Torras, J, Llado, L, Lopez-ben, S, Codina-barreras, A, & Mojal, S. Effect of subcentimeter nonpositive resection margin on hepatic recurrence in patients undergoing hepatectomy for colorectal liver metastases. Evidences from 663 liver resections. Annals of Oncology (2007). , 18, 1190-95.

[39] Lordan, J. T, & Karanjia, N. D. Size of surgical margin does not influence recurrence rates after curative liver resection for colorectal cancer liver metastases. Br J Surg (2007). , 94, 1133-8.

[40] Poultsides, G. A, Schulick, R. D, & Pawlik, T. M. Hepatic resection for colorectal metastases: the impact of surgical margin status on outcome. HPB (2010). , 12, 43-9.

[41] Elias, D, Liberale, G, Vernerey, D, Pocard, M, Ducreux, M, Boige, V, Malka, D, Pignon, J. P, & Lasser, P. Hepatic and extrahepatic colorectal metastases: when resectable, their localization does not matter, but their total number has a prognostic effect. Ann Surg Oncol (2005). , 12, 900-9.

[42] Elias, D, Ouellet, J. F, & Bellon, N. Extrahepatic disease does not contraindicate hepatectomy for colorectal liver metastases. Br J Surg (2003). , 90, 567-74.

[43] Khatri, V. P, Petrelli, N. J, & Belghiti, J. Extending the frontiers of surgical therapy for hepatic colorectal metastases: is there a limit? J Clin Oncol (2005). , 23, 8490-9.

[44] Minagawa, M, Makuuchi, M, Torzilli, G, Takayama, T, Kawasaki, S, Kosuge, T, Yamamoto, J, & Imamura, H. Extension of the frontiers of surgical indications in the treatment of liver metastases from colorectal cancer: long-term results. Ann Surg (2000). , 231, 487-99.

[45] Kanemitsu, Y, Kato, T, Hirai, T, & Yasui, K. Preoperative probability model for predicting overall survival after resection of pulmonary metastases from colorectal cancer. Br J Surg (2004). , 91, 112-20.

[46] Vauthey, J. N. Colorectal Liver Metastases: Treat Effectively Up Front and Consider the Borderline Resectable. J Clin Oncol (2007). , 25(29), 4524-5.

[47] Adam, R, De Haas, R. J, Wicherts, D. A, Aloia, T. A, Delvart, V, Azoulay, D, Bismuth, H, & Castaing, D. Is hepatic resection justified after chemotherapy in patients with colorectal liver metastases and lymph node involvement? J Clin Oncol (2008). , 26(22), 3672-80.

[48] Jaeck, D. The significance of hepatic pedicle lymph nodes metastases in surgical management of colorectal liver metastases and of other liver malignancies. Ann Surg Oncol (2003). , 10, 1007-11.

[49] Lehmann, K, & Rickenbacher, A. AWeber, Pestalozzi BC, Clavien PA. Chemotherapy Before Liver Resection of Colorectal Metastases: Friend or Foe? Ann Surg (2012). , 255(2), 237-47.

[50] Nondlinger, B, Sorbye, H, Glimelius, B, Poston, G. J, Schlag, P. M, Rougier, P, Bechstein, W. O, Primrose, J. N, Walpole, E. T, Finch-jones, M, Jaeck, D, Mirza, D, Parks, R. W, Collette, L, Praet, M, Bethe, U, Van Cutsem, E, Scheithauer, W, & Gruenberger, T. Perioperative chemotherapy with FOLFOX4 and surgery versus surgery alone for resectable liver metastases from colorectal cancer (EORTC Intergroup trial 40983): a randomised controlled trial. Lancet (2008). , 371, 1007-16.

[51] Kooby, D. A, Stockman, J, Ben-porat, L, Gonen, M, Jarnagin, W. R, Dematteo, R. P, Tuorto, S, Wuest, D, Blumgart, L. H, & Fong, Y. Influence of transfusions on perioperative and long-term outcome in patients following hepatic resection for colorectal metastases. Ann Surg (2003). , 237, 860-70.

[52] Strasberg, S. M, Belghiti, J, Clavien, P. A, Gadzijev, E, Garden, J. O, Lau, W. Y, Makuuchi, M, & Strong, R. W. Terminology Committee of the International Hepato-Pancreato-Biliary Association: The Brisbane 2000 Terminology of Liver Anatomy and Resections. HPB (2000). , 2, 333-9.

[53] De Haas, R. J, Wicherts, D. A, Flores, E, Azoulay, D, Castaing, D, & Adam, R. R. resection by necessity for colorectal liver metastases: Is it still a contraindication to surgery? Ann Surg (2008). , 248(4), 626-37.

[54] Gagner, M, Rheault, M, & Dubuc, J. Laparoscopic partial hepatectomy for liver tumour. Surg Endosc (1992).

[55] Cellini, C, Hunt, S. R, Fleshman, J. W, Birnbaum, E. H, Bierhals, A. J, & Mutch, M. G. Stage IV rectal cancer with liver metastases: is there a benefit to resection of the primary tumour? World J Surg (2010). , 34(5), 1102-8.

[56] Adam, R, Delvart, V, Pascal, G, Castaing, D, Azoulay, D, Giacchetti, S, Paule, B, Kunstlinger, F, Ghémard, O, Levi, F, & Bismuth, H. Rescue surgery for unresectable colorectal liver metastases downstaged by chemotherapy: a model to predict long-term survival. Ann Surg (2004). , 240, 644-57.

[57] Benoist, S, Brouquet, A, Penna, C, Julié, C, El Hajjam, M, Chagnon, S, Mitry, E, Rougier, P, & Nordlinger, B. Complete response of colorectal liver metastases after chemotherapy: does it mean cure? J Clin Oncol (2006). , 20(24), 3939-45.

[58] Abdalla, E. K, Adam, R, Bilchik, A. J, Jaeck, D, Vauthey, J. N, & Mahvi, R. Improving resectability of hepatic colorectal metastases: Expert consensus statement. Annals of Surgical Oncology (2006). , 13(10), 1271-80.

[59] Donadon, M, Ribero, D, Morris-stiff, G, Abdalla, E. K, & Vauthey, J. N. New paradigm in the management of liver-only metastases from colorectal cancer. Gastrointest Cancer Res (2007). , 1(1), 20-7.

[60] Garden, O. J, Rees, M, Poston, G. J, Mirza, D, Saunders, M, Ledermann, J, Primrose, J. N, & Parks, R. W. Guidelines for resection of colorectal cancer liver metastases. Gut (2006). Suppl 3): iiiiii8., 1.

[61] De Haas, R J, Wicherts, D. A, Andreani, P, Pascal, G, Saliba, F, Ichai, P, Adam, R, Castaing, D, & Azoulay, D. Impact of expanding criteria for resectability of colorectal metastases on short- and long-term outcomes after hepatic resection. Ann Surg (2011). , 253(6), 1069-79.

[62] Power, D. G, & Kemeny, N. E. Role of adjuvant therapy after resection of colorectal cancer liver metastases. J Clin Oncol (2010). , 28(13), 2300-9.

[63] Laurent, C. Sa Cunha A, Couderc P, Rullier E, Saric J. Influence of postoperative morbidity on long-term survival following liver resection for colorectal metastases. Br J Surg (2003). , 90(9), 1131-6.

[64] Makuuchi, M, Thai, B. L, Takayasu, K, Takayama, T, Kosuge, T, Gunven, P, Yamazaki, S, Hasegawa, H, & Ozaki, H. Preoperative portal embolization to increase safety of major hepatectomy for hilar bile duct carcinoma: a preliminary report. Surgery (1990). , 107, 521-7.

[65] Ribero, D, Abdallah, E. K, Madoff, D. C, Donadon, M, Loyer, E. M, & Vauthey, J. N. Portal vein embolization before major hepatectomy and its effects on regeneration, resectability and outcome. Br J Surg (2007). , 94, 1386-96.

[66] Abdallah, E. K, Hicks, M. E, & Vauthey, J. N. Portal vein embolization: rationale, technique and future prospects. Br J Surg (2001). , 88, 165-75.

[67] Nagino, M, Kamiya, J, Nishio, H, Ebata, T, Arai, T, & Nimura, Y. Two hundred forty consecutive portal vein embolizations before extended hepatectomy for biliary cancer: surgical outcome and long-term follow-up. Ann Surg (2006). , 243, 364-72.

[68] Azoulay, D, Castaing, D, Smail, A, Adam, R, Cailliez, V, Laurent, A, Lemoine, A, & Bismuth, H. Resection of non-resectable liver metastases from colorectal cancer after percutaneous portal vein embolization. Ann Surg (2000). , 4, 480-86.

[69] Adam, R, Laurent, A, Azoulay, D, Castaing, D, & Bismuth, H. Two-stage hepatectomy: a planned strategy to treat irresectable liver tumours. Ann Surg (2000). , 232, 777-85.

[70] Jaeck, D, Oussoultzoglou, E, Rosso, E, Greget, M, Weber, J. C, & Bachellier, P. Two-stage hepatectomy procedure combined with portal vein embolization to achieve curative resection for initially unresectable multiple and bilobar colorectal liver metastases. Ann Surg (2004). , 240, 1037-49.

[71] Clavien, P. A, Petrowsky, H, Deoliveira, M. L, & Graf, R. Strategies for safer liver surgery and partial liver transplantation. N Engl J Med (2007). , 356(15), 1545-59.

[72] Kianmanesh, R, Farges, O, Abdalla, E. K, & Sauvanet, A. Ruszniewski, Belghiti J. Right portal vein ligation: a new planned two-step all-surgical approach for complete resection of primary gastrointestinal tumours with multiple bilateral liver metastases. J Am Coll Surg (2003). , 197, 164-70.

[73] Brouquet, A, Abdalla, E. K, Kopetz, S, Garrett, C. R, Overman, M. J, Eng, C, Andreou, A, Loyer, E. M, Madoff, D. C, Curley, S. A, & Vauthey, J. N. High survival rate after two-stage resection of advanced colorectal liver metastases: responsebased selection and complete resection define outcome. J Clin Oncol (2011). , 29, 1083-90.

[74] Narita, M, Oussoultzoglou, E, Jaeck, D, Fuchschuber, P, Rosso, E, Pessaux, P, Marzano, E, & Bachellier, P. Two-stage hepatectomy for multiple bilobar colorectal liver metastases. Br J Surg (2011). , 98(10), 1463-75.

[75] Schnitzbauer, A. A, Lang, S. A, Goessmann, H, Nadalin, S, Baumgart, J, Farkas, S. A, Fichtner-feigl, S, Lorf, T, Goralcyk, A, Hörbelt, R, Kroemer, A, Loss, M, Rümmele, P, Scherer, M. N, Padberg, W, Königsrainer, A, Lang, H, Obed, A, & Schlitt, H. J. Right Portal Vein Ligation Combined With In Situ Splitting Induces Rapid Left Lateral Liver Lobe Hypertrophy Enabling 2-Staged Extended Right Hepatic Resection in Small-for-Size Settings. Ann Surg (2012). , 255(3), 405-14.

[76] Andriani, O. C. Long-Term Results With ssociating Liver Partition and Portal Vein Ligation for Staged Hepatectomy (ALPPS). Annals of Surgery (2012). e5.

[77] Clavien-3, P. A, & Santibañes, E. The ALPPS: Time to Explore! Ann Surg (2012). e, 18-9.

[78] Machado MACMakdissi FF, Surjan RC. Totally Laparoscopic ALPPS Is Feasible and May Be Worthwhile. Annals of Surgery (2012). e13.

[79] Conrad, C, Shivathirthan, N, Camerlo, A, Strauss, C, & Gayet, B. Laparoscopic Portal Vein Ligation With In Situ Liver Split for Failed Portal Vein Embolization. Annals of Surgery (2012). e, 14-5.

[80] Aloia, T. A, & Vauthey, J. N. Associating Liver Partition and Portal Vein Ligation for Staged Hepatectomy (ALPPS): What Is Gained and What Is Lost? Annals of Surgery (2012). e9.

[81] Jain, H. A. Bharathy KGS, Negi SS. Associating Liver Partition and Portal Vein Ligation for Staged Hepatectomy: Will the Morbidity of an Additional Surgery Be Outweighed by Better Patient Outcomes in the Long-Term? Annals of Surgery (2012). e10.

[82] Narita, M, Oussoultzoglou, E, Ikai, I, Bachellier, P, & Jaeck, D. Right Portal Vein Ligation Combined With In Situ Splitting Induces Rapid Left Lateral Liver Lobe Hyper-

trophy Enabling Staged Extended Right Hepatic Resection in Small-for-Size Settings. Annals of Surgery (2012 2). e7-8., 2.

[83] Dokmak, S, & Belghiti, J. Which limits to the "ALPPS" Approach? Annals of Surgery (2012). e6.

[84] Santibañes, E, & Clavien, P. A. Playing Play-Doh to Prevent Postoperative Liver Failure: The "ALPPS" approach. Annals of Surgery (2012). , 256(3), 415-7.

[85] Konopke, R, Roth, J, Volk, A, Pistorius, S, Folprecht, G, Zoephel, K, Schuetze, C, Laniado, M, Saeger, H. D, & Kersting, S. Colorectal Liver Metastases: an Update on Palliative Treatment Options. J Gastrointestin Liver Dis (2012). , 21(1), 83-91.

[86] Solbiati, L, Livraghi, T, Goldberg, S. N, et al. Percutaneous radiofrequency ablation of hepatic metastases from colorectal cancer: long-term results in 117 patients. Radiology (2001). , 221, 159-66.

[87] Sorensen, S. M, Mortensen, F. V, & Nielsen, D. T. Radiofrequency ablation of colorectal liver metastases: long-term survival. Acta Radiol (2007). , 48, 253-8.

[88] Machi, J, Oishi, A. J, Sumida, K, Sakamoto, K, Furumoto, N. L, Oishi, R. H, & Kylstra, J. W. Long-term outcome of radiofrequency ablation for unresectable liver metastases from colorectal cancer: evaluation of prognostic factors and effectiveness in first- and second-line management. Cancer J (2006). , 12, 318-26.

[89] Kennedy, J. E. High-intensity focused ultrasound in the treatment of solid tumours. Nat Rev Cancer (2005). , 5, 321-7.

[90] Al-asfoor, A, Federowicz, Z, & Lodge, M. Resection versus no intervention or other surgical interventions for colorectal cancer liver metastases. Cochrane Database Syst Rev (2008). CD006039.

[91] Azoulay, D, Eshkenazy, R, Andreani, P, Castaing, D, Adam, R, Ichai, P, Naili, S, Vinet, E, Saliba, F, Lemoine, A, Gillon, M. C, & Bismuth, H. In situ hypothermic perfusion of the liver versus standard total vascular exclusion of complex liver resection. Ann Surg (2005). , 2005, 241-277.

[92] Hemming, A. W, Chari, R. S, & Cattral, M. S. Ex vivo liver resection. Can J Surg (2000). , 43(3), 222-4.

[93] Lodge JPAAmmori BJ, Prasad KR, Bellamy MC. Ex vivo and in situ resection of inferior vena cava with hepatectomy for colorectal metastases. Ann Surg (2000). , 231(4), 471-9.

[94] Hemming, A. W, & Reed, A. I. Langham MR Jr, Fujita S, Howard RJ. Combined resection of the liver and inferior vena cava for hepatic malignancy. Ann Surg (2004). , 239, 712-21.

[95] Langenhoff, B. S, Krabbe, P. F, & Ruers, T. J. Efficacy of follow-up after surgical treatment of colorectal liver metastases. Eur J Surg Oncol (2009). , 35, 180-6.

[96] Petrelli, N. Perioperative or adjuvant therapy for resectable colorectal hepatic metastases. J Clin Oncol (2008). , 26(30), 4862-3.

[97] Smith, M. D, & Mccall, J. L. Systematic review of tumour number and outcome after radical treatment of colorectal liver metastases. Br J Surg (2009). , 96(10), 1101-13.

[98] Söreide, J. A, Eiriksson, K, Sandvik, O, Viste, A, Horn, A, Johnsen, G, & Grønbech, J. E. Surgical treatment of liver metastases from colorectal cancer. Br J Surg (2008). , 128, 50-3.

[99] Petrowsky, H, Gonen, M, Jarnagin, W, Lorenz, M, Dematteo, R, Heinrich, S, Encke, A, Blumgart, L, & Fong, Y. Second liver resections are safe and effective treatment for recurrent hepatic metastases from colorectal cancer: a bi- institutional analysis. Ann Surg (2002). , 235, 863-71.

[100] Yamamoto, J, Kosuge, T, Shimada, K, Yamasaki, S, Moriya, Y, & Sugihara, K. Repeat liver resection for recurrent colorectal liver metastases. Am J Surg (1999). , 178, 275-81.

[101] Adam, R, Pascal, G, Azoulay, D, Tanaka, K, Castaing, D, & Bismuth, H. Liver resection for colorectal metastases: the third hepatectomy. Ann Surg (2005). , 238, 871-83.

[102] International Agency for Research on Cancer: GLOBOCAN 2008 dataWorld Health Organization. Cancer Incidence, Mortality and Prevalence Worldwide in (2008). http://www-dep.iarc.fraccessed 22 August 2012)

[103] Borrego-Estella, V. M, & Serrablo, A. In: Borrego-Estella VM (ed.) Estudio de las metástasis hepáticas de cáncer colorrectal con rescate quirúrgico en un hospital de tercer nivel. Identificación de marcadores biológicos pronósticos. Salamanca: Colección VITOR; (2010). , 12-19.

[104] Berge, T, & Linell, F. Carcinoid tumours. Frequency in defined population during a 12-year period. Acta Pathol Microbiol Scand (1976). , 84(4), 322-30.

[105] Hellman, P, Lundström, T, Öhrvall, U, Eriksson, B, Skogseid, B, & Oberg, K. Tiensuu Janson E, Akerstrom G. Effect of surgery on the outcome of midgut carcinoid disease with lymph node and liver metastases. World J Surg (2002). , 26, 991-7.

[106] Touzius, J. G, Kiely, J. M, Pitt, S. C, Rilling, W. S, Quebbeman, E. J, Wilson, S. D, & Pitt, H. Neuroendocrine hepatic metastases: does aggressive management improve survival? Ann Surg (2005). , 241(5), 776-83.

[107] Hodul, P, Malafa, M, Choi, J, & Kvols, L. The role of cytoreductive hepatic surgery as an adjunct to the management of metastatic neuorendocrine carcinomas. Cancer Control (2006). , 13, 61-71.

[108] Lee PSYCheow PC, Teo JY, Ooi LLPJ. Surgical treatment of neuroendocrine liver metastases. Int J Hepatol (2012). Epub 2012 Jan 26.

[109] Steinmueller, T, Kianmanesh, R, Falconi, M, Scarpa, A, Taal, B, Kuekkeboom, D. J, Lopes, J. M, Perren, A, & Nikou, G. Delle Fave GF, O'Toole D, Frascati Concensus

Conference Participants: Consensus guidelines for the management of patients with liver metastases from digestive (neuro)endocrine tumours: foregut, midgut, hindgut, and unknown primary. Neuroendocrinology (2008). , 87, 47-62.

[110] Sarmiento, J. M, Heywood, G, Rubin, J, Ilstrup, D. M, Nagorney, D. M, & Qne, F. G. Surgical treatment of neuroendocrine metastases to the liver: a plea for resection to increase survival. J Am Coll Surg (2003). , 197, 29-37.

[111] Knox, C. D, Anderson, C. D, Lamps, L. W, Adkins, R. B, & Pinson, C. W. Long-term survival after resection for primary hepatic carcinoid tumour. Ann Surg Oncol (2003). , 10(10), 1171-5.

[112] Musunuru, S, Chen, H, Rajpal, S, Stephani, N, Mcdermott, J. C, Holen, K, Rikkers, L. F, & Weber, S. M. Metastatic neuroendocrine hepatic tumours: resection improves survival. Arch Surg (2006). , 141, 1000-4.

[113] Frilling, A, Rogiers, X, Malago, M, Liedke, O. M, Kaun, M, & Broelsch, C. E. Treatment of liver metastases in patients with neuroendocrine tumours. Langenbeck 's Arch Surg (1998). , 383, 62-70.

[114] Adam, R, Chiche, L, Aloia, T, Elias, D, Salmon, R, Rivoire, M, Jaeck, D, & Saric, J. Le-Treut YP, Belghiti J, Mantion G, Mentha G and the Association Française de Chirurgie. Hepatic resection for noncolorectal nonendocrine liver metastases. Analysis of 1452 patients and development of a prognostic model. Ann Surg (2006). , 244(4), 524-35.

[115] Reddy, S. K, Barbas, A. S, Marroquin, C. E, Morse, M. A, Kuo, P. C, & Clary, B. M. Resection of noncolorectal nonneuroendocrine liver metastases: a comparative analysis. J Am Coll Surg (2007). , 204, 372-82.

[116] Harrison, L. E, Brennan, M. F, Newman, E, Fortner, J. G, Picardo, A, & Blumgart, L. H. Hepatic resection for noncolorectal, nonneuroendocrine metastases: a fifteen-year experience with ninety-six patients. Surgery (1997). , 121, 625-32.

[117] Hemming, A. W, Sielaff, T. D, Gallinger, S, Cattral, M. S, Taylor, B. R, Greig, P. D, & Langer, B. Hepatic resection of noncolorectal nonneuroendocrine metastases. Liver Transpl (2000). , 6, 97-101.

[118] Laurent, C, Rullier, E, Feyler, A, Masson, B, & Saric, J. Resection of noncolorectal and nonneuroendocrine liver metastases: late meatastases are the only chance of cure. World J Surg (2001). , 25, 1532-6.

[119] Yamada, H, Katoh, H, Kondo, S, Okushiba, S, & Morikawa, T. Hepatectomy from non-colorectal and non-neuroendocrine tumour. Anticancer Res (2001). , 21, 4159-62.

[120] Takada, Y, Otsuka, M, Seino, K, Taniguchi, H, Koike, N, Kawamoto, T, Koda, K, Adachi, S, Yuzawa, K, Nozue, M, Todoroki, T, & Fukao, K. Hepatic resection for metastatic tumours from noncolorectal carcinoma. Hepatogastroenterology. (2001). , 48, 83-6.

[121] Karavias, D. D, Tepetes, K, Karatzas, T, Felekouras, E, & Androulakis, J. Liver resection for metastatic non-olorectal non-neuroendocrine hepatic neoplasms. Eur J Surg Oncol (2002). , 28, 135-9.

[122] Weitz, J, Blumgart, L. H, Fong, Y, Jarnagin, W. R, Angelica, D, Harrison, M, & Dematteo, L. E. RP. Partial hepatectomy for metastases from noncolorectal, nonneuroendocrine carcinoma. Ann Surg (2005). , 241, 269-76.

[123] Ercolani, G, Grazi, G. L, Ravaioli, M, Ramacciato, G, Cescon, M, & Varotti, G. del Gaudio M, Vetrone G, Pinna AD. The role of liver resections for oncolorectal, nonneuroendocrine metastases: experience with 142 observed cases. Ann Surg Oncol (2005). , 12, 459-66.

[124] Miettinen, M, & Lasota, J. Gastrointestinal stromal tumours: definition, clinical, histological, immunohistochemical, and molecular genetic features and differential diagnosis. Virchows Arch (2001). , 438, 1-12.

[125] Gold, J. S. DeMatteo RP: Combined surgical and medical therapy, the gastrointestinal stromal tumour model. Ann Surg (2006). , 244, 176-84.

[126] Miettinen, M, Rifai, W, Sobin, H. L, & Lasota, L. J. Evaluation of malignancy and prognosis of gastrointestinal stromal tumours: a review. Hum Pathol (2002). , 33, 478-83.

[127] Gomez, D, Al-mukthar, A, Menon, K. V, Toogood, G. J, Lodge, J. P, & Prasad, K. R. Aggressive surgical resection for the management of hepatic metastases from gastrointestinal stromal tumours: a single centre experience. HPB (2007). , 9, 64-70.

[128] Dematteo, R. P, Lewis, J. J, Leung, D, Mudan, S. S, Woodruff, J. M, & Brennan, M. F. Two hundred gastrointestinal stromal tumours: recurrence patterns and prognostic factors for survival. Ann Surg (2000). , 231, 51-8.

[129] Husted, T. L, Neff, G, Thomas, M. J, Gross, T. G, Woodle, E. S, & Buell, J. F. Liver transplantation for primary or metastatic sarcoma to the liver. Am J Transplant (2006). , 6, 392-7.

[130] Turley, R. S, Peng, P. D, Reddy, S. K, Barbas, A. S, Geller, D. A, Marsh, J. W, Tsung, A, Pawlik, T. M, & Clary, B. M. Hepatic resection for metastatic gastrointestinal stromal tumours in the tyrosine kinase inhibitor era. Cancer (2012). , 118(14), 3571-8.

[131] Ng, E. H, Pollock, R. E, Munsell, M. F, Atkinson, E. N, & Romsdahl, M. M. Prognostic factors influencing survival in gastrointestinal leiomyosarcomas. Implications for surgical management and staging. Ann Surg (1992). , 215, 68-77.

[132] Chen, H, Pruitt, A, Nicol, T. L, Gorgulu, S, & Choti, M. A. Complete hepatic resection of metastases from leiomyosarcoma prolongs survival. J Gastrointest Surg (1998). , 2, 151-5.

[133] Lang, H, Nussbaum, K. T, Kaudel, P, Fruhauf, N, Flemming, P, & Raab, R. Hepatic metastases from leiomyosarcoma: a single center experience with 34 liver resections during a 15-year period. Ann Surg (2000). , 231, 500-5.

[134] Shima, Y, Horimi, T, Ishikawa, T, Ichikawa, J, Okabayashi, T, Nishioka, Y, Hamada, M, Shibuya, Y, Ishii, T, & Ito, M. Aggressive surgery for liver metastases from gastrointestinal stromal tumours. J Hepatobiliary Pancreat Surg (2003). , 10, 77-80.

[135] Nunobe, S, Sano, T, Shimada, K, Sakamoto, Y, & Kosuge, T. Surgery including liver resection for metastatic gastrointestinal stromal tumours or gastrointestinal leiomyosarcomas. Jpn J Clin Oncol (2005). , 35, 338-41.

[136] Seifert, J. K, Weigel, T. F, Gonner, U, Bottger, T. C, & Junginger, T. Liver resection for breast cancer metastases. Hepatogastroenterology (1999). , 46, 2935-40.

[137] Atalay, G, Biganzoli, L, Renard, F, Paridaens, R, Cufer, T, Coleman, R, Calvert, A. H, Gamucci, T, Minisini, A, Therasse, P, & Piccart, M. J. Clinical outcome of breast cancer patients with liver metastases alone in the anthracycline-taxane era: A retrospective analysis of two prospective, randomised metastatic breast cancer trials. Eur J Cancer (2003). , 39, 2439-49.

[138] Adam, R, Aloia, T, Krissat, J, Bralet, M. P, Paule, B, Gachietti, S, Delvart, S, Azoulay, D, Bismuth, H, & Castaing, D. Is liver resection justified for patients with hepatic metastases from breast cancer? Ann Surg (2006). , 244, 897-908.

[139] Elias, D, Maisonnette, F, Druet-cabanc, M, Ouellet, J. F, Guinebretiere, J. M, Spielmann, M, & Delaloge, S. An attempt to clarify indications for hepatectomy for liver metastases from breast cancer. Am J Surg (2003). , 185, 158-64.

[140] Weitz, J, Blumgart, L. H, Fong, Y, Jarnagin, W. R, Angelica, D, Harrison, M, & Dematteo, L. E. RP. Partial hepatectomy for metastases from noncolorectal nonneuroendocrine carcinoma. Ann Surg (2005). , 241, 269-76.

[141] Sakamoto, Y, Yamamoto, J, Yoshimoto, M, & Kasumi, F. Kosuge bT, Kokudo N, Makuuchi M. Hepatic resection for metastatic breast cancer: prognostic analysis of 34 patients. World J Surg (2005). , 29, 524-7.

[142] Carlini, M, Lonardo, M. T, Carboni, F, Petric, M, Vitucci, C, Santoro, R, & Lepiane, P. Liver metastases from breast cancer: Results of surgical resection. Hepatogastroenterology (2002). , 49, 597-601.

[143] Yoshimoto, M, Tada, T, Saito, M, Takahashi, K, Uchida, Y, & Kasumi, F. Surgical treatment of hepatic metastases from breast cancer. Breast Cancer Res Treat (2000). , 59, 177-84.

[144] Selzner, M, Morse, M. A, Vredenburgh, J. J, Meyers, W. C, & Clavien, P. A. Liver metastases from breast cancer: long-term survival after curative resection. Surgery (2000). , 127, 383-9.

[145] Pocard, M, Pouillart, P, Asselain, B, Falcou, M. C, & Salmon, R. J. Resections hepatiques pour metastases de cancer du sein: resultats et facteurs pronostiques (65 cas). Ann Chir (2001). , 126, 413-20.

[146] Raab, R, Nussbaum, K. T, Werner, U, & Pichlmayr, R. Liver metastases in breast carcinoma. Results of partial liver resection. Chirurg (1996). , 67, 234-7.

[147] Scheuerlein, H, Schneider, C, Köckerling, F, & Hohenberger, W. Surgical therapy of liver metastases in breast carcinoma]. Zentralbl Chir (1998). Suppl , 5, 130-4.

[148] Pawlik, T. M, Zorzi, D, Abdalla, E. K, Clary, B. M, Gershenwald, J. E, Ross, M. I, Aloia, T. A, Curley, S. A, Camacho, L. H, Capussotti, L, Elias, D, & Vauthey, J. N. Hepatic resection for metastatic melanoma: distinct patterns of recurrence and prognosis for ocular versus cutaneous disease. Ann Surg Oncol (2006). , 13, 712-20.

[149] Rose, D. M, Essner, R, & Hughes, T. M. Tang PCY, Bilchik A, Wanek LA, Thompson JF, Morton DL. Surgical resection for metastatic melanoma to the liver: the John Wayne Cancer Institute and Sydney Melanoma Unit experience. Arch Surg (2001). , 136, 950-5.

[150] Fuster, D, Chiang, S, Johnson, G, Schuchter, L. M, Zhuang, H, & Alavi, A. Is 18FDG PET more accurate than standard diagnostic procedure in the detection of suspected recurrent melanoma? J Nul Med (2004). , 45, 1323-7.

[151] Stoelben, E, Sturm, J, Schmoll, J, Keilholz, U, & Saeger, H. D. Resection of solitary liver metastases of malignant melanoma. Chirurg (1995). , 66, 40-3.

[152] Wood, T. F. DiFronzo LA, Rose DM, Haigh PI, Stern SL, Wanek L. Does complete resection of melanoma metastatic to solid intra-abdominal organs improve survival? Ann Surg Oncol (2001). , 8, 658-62.

[153] Chua, T. C, Saxena, A, & Morris, D. L. Surgical metastasectomy in AJCC Stage IV M1c melanoma patients with gastrointestinal and liver metastases. Ann Acad Med Singapore (2010). , 39, 634-9.

[154] Essner, R, Lee, J. H, Wanek, L. A, Itakura, H, & Morton, D. L. Contemporary surgical treatment of advanced-stage melanoma. Arch Surg (2004). , 139, 961-7.

[155] Ripley, R. T, Davis, J. L, Klapper, J. A, Mathur, A, Kammula, U, Royal, R. E, Yang, J. C, Sherry, R. M, Hughes, M. S, Libutti, S. K, White, D. E, Steinberg, S. M, Dudley, M. E, Rosenberg, S. A, & Avital, I. Liver resection for melanoma with postoperative tumour-inflitrating lymphocyte therapy. Ann Surg Oncol (2010). , 17(1), 163-70.

[156] Herman, P. Machado MAC, Montagnini AL, Albuquerque LA, Saad WA, Machado MC. Selected patients with metastatic melanoma may benefit from liver resction. World J Surg (2007). , 31, 171-4.

[157] Crook, T. B. Jones Om, John TG, Rees M. Hepatic resection for malignan melanoma. Eur J Surg Oncol , 20032, 315-7.

[158] Sakamoto, Y, Ohyama, S, Yamamoto, J, Yamada, K, Seki, M, Ohta, K, Kokudo, N, Yamaguchi, T, Muto, T, & Makuuchi, M. Surgical resection of liver metastases of gastric cancer: an analysis of a 17-year experience with 22 patients. Surgery (2003). , 133, 507-11.

[159] Thelen, A, Jonas, S, Benckert, C, Lopez-hänninen, E, Neumann, U, Rudolph, B, Schumacher, G, & Neuhaus, P. Liver resection for metastatic gastric cancer. Eur J Surg Oncol (2008). , 34(12), 1328-34.

[160] Shirabe, K, Shimada, M, Matsumata, T, Higashi, H, Yakeishi, Y, & Wakiyama, S. Analysis of the prognostic factors for liver metastasis of gastric cancer after hepatic resection: a multiinstitutional study of the indications for resection. Hepatogastroenterology (2003). , 50, 1560-3.

[161] Ambiru, S, Miyazaki, M, Ito, H, Nakagawa, K, Shimizu, H, Yoshidome, H, Shimizu, Y, & Nakajima, N. Benefits and limits of hepatic resection for gastric metastases. Am J Surg (2001). , 181, 279-83.

[162] Zacherl, J, Zacherl, M, Scheuba, C, Steininger, R, Wenzl, E, Muhlbacher, F, Jakesz, R, & Längle, F. Analysis of hepatic resection of metastasis originating from gastric adenocarcinoma. J Gastrointest Surg (2002). , 6, 682-9.

[163] Saiura, A, Umekita, N, Inoue, S, Maeshiro, T, Miyamoto, S, Matsui, Y, Asakage, t, & Kitamura, M. M. Clinicopathological features and outcome of hepatic resection for liver metastasis from gastric cancer. Hepatogastroenterology (2002). , 49, 1062-5.

[164] Okano, K, Maeba, T, Ishimura, K, Karasawa, Y, Goda, F, Wakabayashi, H, Usuki, H, & Maeta, H. Hepatic resection for metastatic tumours from gastric cancer. Ann Surg , 2002235, 86-91.

[165] Roh, H. R, Suh, K. S, Lee, H. J, Yang, H. K, Choe, K. J, & Lee, K. U. Outcome of hepatic resection for metastatic gastric cancer. Am Surg (2005). , 71, 95-9.

[166] Lindell, G, Ohlsson, B, Saarela, A, Andersson, R, & Tranberg, K. G. Liver resection of noncolorectal secondaries. J Surg Oncol (1998). , 69, 66-70.

[167] Di Carlo IGrasso G, Patane D, Russello D, Latteri F. Liver metastases from lung cancer: is surgical resection justified? Ann Thorac Surg (2003). , 76, 291-3.

[168] Ercolani, G, Ravaioli, M, Grazi, G. L, Cescon, M, & Varotti, G. Del Gaudio M, Vetrone G, Zanello M, Principe A, Pinna AD. The role of liver resections for metastases from lung carcinoma. HPB (Oxford) (2006). , 8(2), 114-5.

[169] Armstrong, D. K, Bundy, B, Wenzel, L, & Huang, H. Q. Baergen MSR, Lele S, Copeland LJ, Walker JL, Burger RA. Intraperitoneal cisplatin and paclitaxel in ovarian cancer. N Engl J Med (2006). , 354(5), 34-43.

[170] Yoon, S. S, Jarnagin, W. R, Fong, Y, Dematteo, R. P, Barakat, R. R, Blumgart, L. H, & Chi, D. S. Resection of recurrent ovarian or fallopipan tube carcinoma involving the liver. Gynecol Oncol , 200391, 383-8.

[171] Rasco, D. W. Assikis, Marshall F. Integrating metastasectomy in the managemente of advance urological malignancies-when are we in 2005? J Urol (2006). , 176, 1921-6.

[172] Alves, A, Adam, R, Majno, P, Delvart, V, Azoulay, D, Castaing, D, & Bismuth, H. Hepatic resection for metastatic renal tumours: is it worthwhile? Ann Surg Oncol (2003). , 10, 705-10.